# SEX SENSE
## CANADIAN CONTRACEPTION GUIDE
SECOND, REVISED EDITION

# PREFACE
## AND ACKNOWLEDGEMENTS

We believe that contraception is a very important key to not only sexual health, but to health and happiness in general. This book is a practical guide on how to be safely sexual as one student who worked on the development of the book put it: "How to have a blast while staying out of trouble!"

You may ask yourself why the SOGC decided to publish a book on contraception. You have probably already seen a variety of pamphlets and brochures on this subject. We felt that we should share with you the experience and knowledge we have as a medical organization. Canadians who want to learn more about their health and about the choices they have to stay healthy should have access to a professional and complete source of information.

The text is based on the Canadian Consensus Conference on Contraception. What is that? Medical professionals with a special interest in sexual health from across Canada got together and came up with guidelines to help other health care professionals serve you better. These guidelines were published in 2004. They are based on evidence, the results of clinical studies. These guidelines can be accessed on our website at www.sogc.org (under publications/guidelines/gynaecology).

This book is about everything you will ever want to know about contraception. Each method is presented in a question and answer format. Included are important questions like, "How effective is a chosen method in preventing pregnancy and sexually transmitted infections and HIV?"

This guide should support you in choosing a contraceptive method that best suits your health and lifestyle.

We owe thanks to the members and chairs of the Contraception Consensus Committee, who provided the groundwork for the manuscript.

Special thanks to the many people who helped to make this book possible:
- A design team from the Design Art Department of Concordia University in Montreal (four dedicated and skilled students and their professor) created the original artistic part of what you have in your hands now.
- The people who took the time and patience to revise the entire manuscript. Thank you for all the comments, advice and great suggestions.
- Thanks also to the many people who provided input on individual chapters.

Throughout the book we present some statistics which give you an idea of what's happening in Canada in terms of contraception and sexual behaviour.
- The 2002 Canadian Contraception Study is a self-report survey, which included 1582 returned questionnaires from women across Canada. They were asked about their choice and satisfaction with contraceptive methods. This study was published in the Journal of Obstetrics Gynaecology Canada in June of 2004 (J Obstet Gynaecol Can. 2004;26:580-90 and J Obstet Gynaecol Can. 2004;26:646-56.)
- The "2004 Global Sex Survey Report" focuses on youths and represents the results of an internet-based survey, which included 350,000 respondents from 41 countries. The report can be viewed on the internet at www.durex.com

The efficacy rates for all contraceptives methods stated in this book are from the following publication: Trussell J. Contraceptive efficacy. In Hatcher RA, Trussell J, Stewart F, Nelson A, Cates W, Guest F, Kowal D. Contraceptive Technology: Eighteens revised edition. New York, NY. Ardent Media 2004.

# INTRODUCTION
## SEX AND HEALTH — ALL ABOUT A WINNING TEAM

**Sex Sense makes sense!**

Since Sex Sense was first published in 2000 much has happened in our country in the contraceptive field! New methods such as the contraceptive patch, the ring and the intrauterine system (IUS) were introduced. Emergency contraception is now available at the pharmacy without a prescription. The SOGC introduced the ultimate Canadian website (sexualityandu.ca) devoted to sexuality education and information. Teens, adults, parents, teachers and health professionals find a wealth of information available 24/7!

**A winning formula**

This book's first edition with a print-run of 100,000 copies has been so popular that we decided to publish a second, revised edition. Sex Sense won the first prize for best book design from Applied Arts Magazine and we got rave reviews from media and readers. Why change a winning formulary? We kept the layout and the table of contents and focused on what's new.

The 2002 Canadian Contraception Study revealed that the main criteria for choosing a method are effectiveness and ease of use. The most popular methods in Canada are oral contraceptives (OCs) (used by 32%), condoms (21%), vasectomy (15%), tubal ligation (8%) and, surprisingly, withdrawal (6%)! Choosing and starting a method is one thing, continuing and being consistent in its use is another. Sex Sense is there to help!

**Sex and Health. About a Winning Team.**

Sex can be fun. Let's face it, for some people it is more important than for others. What is true for everybody is that it touches your body and emotions and can affect your health like no other activity. It can make you ecstatic, happy, want to dance on the moon and reach for the stars. Or it can make you sad and it can make you sick. It can also lead to pregnancy! Don't get us wrong here.

Expecting a baby might be the greatest thing for many couples, but it can also mean disaster to others.

**Where did all the fun go?**

Why is it all so complicated? Why can't we just have fun? Simply because it takes two to tango...and because times have changed drastically. In the good old days you felt attracted to somebody and you had sex. No big deal. Nowadays youth grow up with the warning of HIV, sexually transmitted infections (STIs), and sexual violence. Where did all the fun go?

Let us tell you, it can still be there. But fun might need a bit more planning than it used to. This book helps you to stay out of trouble while enjoying the pleasurable side of sex. This handy guide discusses all contraceptive methods available in Canada. We will look at how they work, how effective they are, and how well they protect you from STIs. At the beginning of each chapter there is a summary of the method. If the summary doesn't spark your interest, forget about that chapter and go to the next method.

**Money, money, money**

You will not find information regarding the cost of each method. Here is why. The costs vary by province and by insurance status and so do the dispensing fees charged by pharmacies.

Most of the hormonal methods, including emergency contraception are covered by health insurance plans. If cost is an issue, you can ask your health care provider about the Compassionate Contraceptive Assistance Program, which gives access to some free contraceptive methods in Canada. Surgical methods and long-term methods such as the IUD and the IUS are also often covered by health insurance. If you opt for barrier methods you will usually have to pay out of your own pocket. In this case it is probably a good idea to shop around for best prices. Condoms are widely available and in some places they are free of charge or reasonably priced.

There are many myths about contraception. This book wants to lift the fog and provide you with fact-based information. The text has short paragraphs, some of which are headed by a question. You can select the sections you are interested in and skip the ones that go into too much detail. This guide will help you make an informed choice about contraception. YOU are important. Take care of yourself. Have fun but protect yourself. Stay healthy and be happy and you'll have it all!

### To do "it" is not everything

Most of the stuff we are talking about in this book involves "it", to have intercourse. This should not give the impression that it is the focal point of having sex. There are a million ways to find pleasure, fulfilment and excitement while having sex, be it with intercourse or without. However, since contraception and protection against STIs and HIV are directly related to the exchange of body fluids, we are focusing on this part of sex. That is why we do not talk a whole lot about other ways of showing affection, passion and desire.

Contraception is also about relationships. A relationship can combine love and sex. It can also be loving without being sexual, and it can also be sexual without love being involved. How is your relationship with your partner? Are you talking about sex? How comfortable are you in sharing a responsibility, like the protection against pregnancy? How long do you want to prevent pregnancy? You should spend time thinking about these questions before making choices.

### You have rights. Use them!

Sexuality is a normal expression of life. The choice of a contraceptive method is more than an intellectual choice. It involves feelings towards sexuality, sense of self, your feelings towards your partner and many other emotions. Be responsible and show respect to your partner. Keep a few things in mind when choosing a contraceptive:

- It is your right to protect yourself from pregnancy and diseases.
- It is your right to enjoy yourself.
- It is your right to determine when, with whom, how, and where you want to have sex.
- It is your right to delay sexual activity.
- It is your right to make your own choices.

We also provide you with addresses, websites and phone numbers of where to turn to with questions regarding contraception, STIs, and unplanned pregnancy. Get started, have fun reading and don't forget to write down any questions that you might have. You should discuss them with your health care provider.

This book cannot replace the care and support that you can get from medical professionals when you have a personal appointment. Family planning clinics, family physicians, gynaecologists, pharmacists, and nurses at schools and universities are there for you. The only thing you have to do is to approach them and they will help you.

Here are some figures from the 2002 Canadian Contraception Study:

- The median age in Canada for first intercourse is 16.5 years.
- At age 15: 11% had intercourse. At age 16: 27%, at age 17: 42%, at age 18: 55%.

# TABLE OF CONTENTS

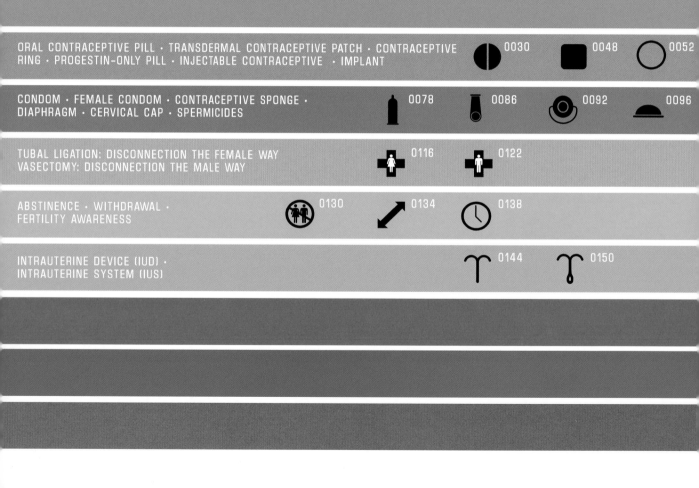

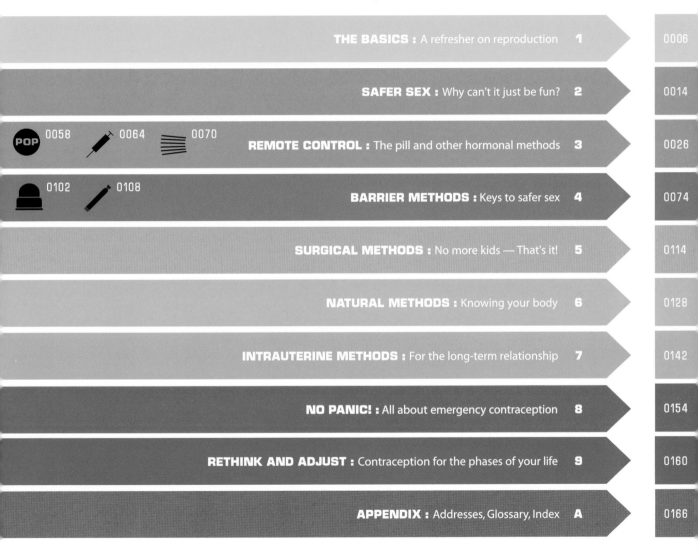

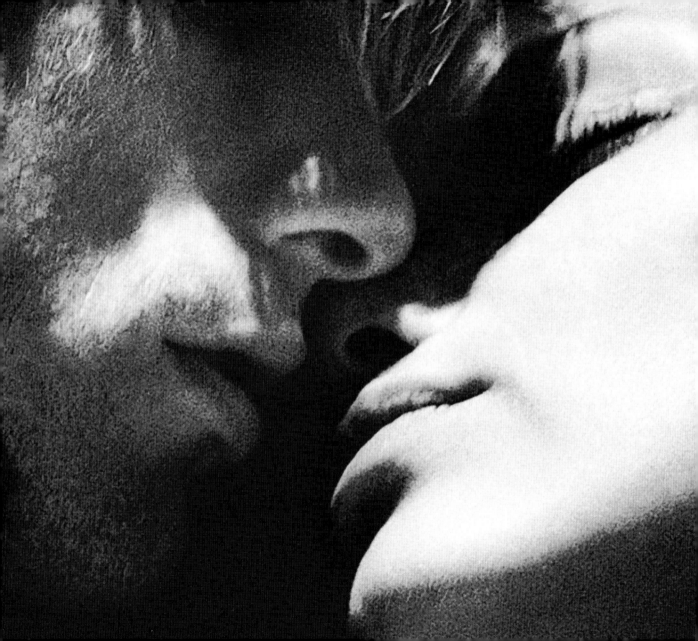

# THE BASICS

## A REFRESHER ON REPRODUCTION

You think you know all about it? Even if you do, here is a refresher course. We will give you some facts on how this business of reproduction works.

Puberty changes the male and female bodies making them physically able to reproduce in order to keep the human race alive. In this book we won't talk about the emotional issues that go along with puberty, however, this is a very exciting time, changing lives forever.

## THE BODY AND THE HORMONES

Most of us are equipped to have kids. Of course there are exceptions, for example when individuals suffer from certain diseases. In addition to organs like the liver, heart, and lungs, we have reproductive organs and we produce hormones inside our bodies. Hormones are courier substances that travel in the blood to carry messages from one organ to another. There are many different types of hormones. One group, sex hormones, controls the ability of women and men to reproduce.

The most important sex hormones in the female body are estrogen and progesterone. The male hormones are called androgens. The most important androgen is testosterone. It is not true that androgens are found only in males and estrogens are found only in females. Men carry female hormones and women carry male hormones as well.

Let's look at the difference between the male and female reproductive organs. When choosing a method of contraception these "little" differences actually make a big difference.

### The male
From the reproductive point of view the major differences between males and females are:
- Starting at puberty, men can make babies basically anytime provided they ejaculate.
- Sperm can stay alive in a woman's reproductive organs for up to three days.
- Men are able to conceive children almost until the end of their lives.
- Men do not have a cycle to regulate fertility like women do.
- Men need to reach orgasm and ejaculate in order to reproduce.

### The sperm production. How men produce babies.
Sperm production begins at the onset of puberty, at an average age of 13 years, and lasts throughout the life of a man. The sure

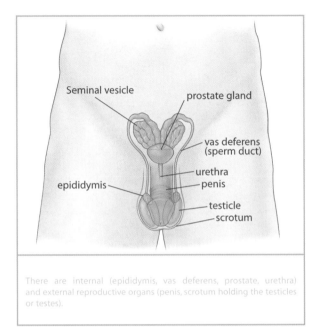

There are internal (epididymis, vas deferens, prostate, urethra) and external reproductive organs (penis, scrotum holding the testicles or testes).

sign for a young man that he is able to reproduce is that his erection is followed by an ejaculation. This is of course only "physically speaking". Emotionally, you might be very far from being ready to take on the responsibility of becoming a father. Sperm, more precisely spermatozoa, are produced by the testicles, which are glands within the scrotum.

The scrotum functions like a thermostat, regulating the temperature of the testicles. If you're a male then you know that the scrotum becomes smaller and more wrinkled when you enter a cold pool. The scrotum contracts to bring the testicles closer to the body to keep them warm. The testicles produce hormones and sperm. Sperm production is an ongoing process. It takes about 70 days for one sperm to mature.

Let's have a look at how sperm actually grow. At the beginning, sperm forms in the testicles, then travels through the epididymis. After that, the sperm reaches the vas deferens. It is stored there until ejaculation occurs. The prostate gland produces a liquid that helps sperm to survive after leaving the male body. During ejaculation, spermatozoa and liquid from the prostate and other glands make a mix while travelling through the urethra. This mix is called semen. The urethra is a tube that also connects to the bladder for passing urine. During sexual excitement, for example during lovemaking, this connection is interrupted so that the semen does not come into contact with urine.

A sperm has the ability to swim and travel on its own. It has an oval-shaped head and a tail that serves as a propeller. Sperm carry the genetic information from the male and can unite with the female egg to produce an embryo. After two months, the embryo becomes a fetus, and later becomes a baby.

### Survival of the fittest
Spermatozoa are very fragile and their chances of survival are very low. This is why the testicles of each individual produce millions of spermatozoa each day. The milky or creamy looking ejaculate consists of hundreds of millions of sperm, but only a few of them will survive the journey through the female vagina to the fallopian tube where the female egg is waiting to meet a sperm. Out of those few, only one will actually penetrate the egg and fertilize it.

Sperm, although it is very fragile, can also be very persistent. Occasionally pregnancy can occur without intercourse and even if the hymen is intact. The hymen is the membrane that partially covers the virgin vagina. This is called "splash pregnancy". Sperm have been known to move very quickly from outside the vagina into the uterus. After intercourse sperm can survive up to three days in the reproductive organs of a female.

### The female
Remember what we said earlier about the differences between the sexes? Here are the little differences that make up a female:

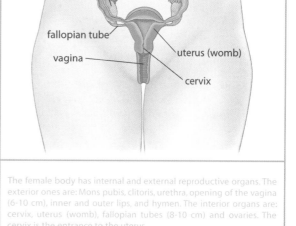

The female body has internal and external reproductive organs. The exterior ones are: Mons pubis, clitoris, urethra, opening of the vagina (6-10 cm), inner and outer lips, and hymen. The interior organs are: cervix, uterus (womb), fallopian tubes (8-10 cm) and ovaries. The cervix is the entrance to the uterus.

- The woman is able to have children from the time she begins to produce eggs (around 12 years) to the onset of menopause (around 52 years).
- The woman can conceive only during the three days (approximately) surrounding ovulation each month (2 days before and on the day of ovulation).
- The woman has a menstrual cycle that determines her fertility.
- The female egg can only be fertilized by male semen in a time period of 6-12 hours.
- The woman can become pregnant without being sexually aroused and reaching orgasm.
- The woman could be a virgin and still get pregnant (splash pregnancy).

## Puberty: when hormones start working overtime

Already at birth, the female body is equipped with a bank account of 300,000-400,000 egg cells, which are located in the ovaries. Of this large amount only 300-500 will be released during the reproductive years of a woman's life. Starting between the ages of 8-10, hormone production rises and makes the body change from a girl to a young woman. The first menstruation, between ages 11-14, is the sure sign that the body is preparing to have children. This is of course only "physically speaking". Emotionally, you might be very far from being ready to have children of your own.

From puberty on:
- The female produces one egg (ovulation) every month in the left or the right ovary.
- This egg is released to start its journey to the uterus through one of the fallopian tubes.
- The body prepares for a possible pregnancy.

Keep in mind that we're talking about the usual stuff here. Of course there are exceptions such as the production of more than one egg, which might lead to two or more babies. This all happens due to the amazing teamwork between the hormones and organs. These things go on over and over again each month and this is what we call the female cycle.

## The amazing female cycle

The cycle covers a time frame of 23-35 days. The average cycle lasts 28 days. The first day of the cycle is the first day of menstruation. The last day of the cycle is the last day before the following menstruation. Cycle lengths vary individually and they are not always regular. Stress, weight gain or weight loss, for example, can disturb it. After the first menstruation it may take 1-3 years until a woman gets a regular cycle.

During the first 14 days of the cycle (usually, but depending on cycle length) an egg is ripening. A hormone in the brain, which is called follicle stimulating hormone (FSH), stimulates the ripening process. The coat around the egg produces estrogen. This most important female hormone makes the lining of the uterus grow to form a nutritious and secure bedding for the egg to settle into after fertilization.

Approximately at day 14 of a 28-day cycle, an egg is ready to be released. Another hormone in the brain, which is called luteinizing hormone (LH), gives the impulse for the egg to emerge from the ovary and be taken up by the fallopian tube. This important event is called ovulation. This is also the most fertile time of the month for the woman to get pregnant. The egg then travels through the fallopian tube to the uterus. The journey takes about seven days. In the meantime, another important hormone produced in the ovary, progesterone, is

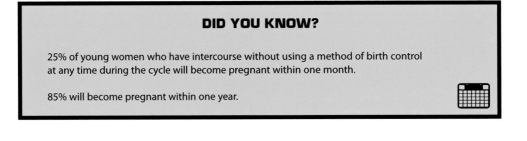

## DID YOU KNOW?

25% of young women who have intercourse without using a method of birth control at any time during the cycle will become pregnant within one month.

85% will become pregnant within one year.

preparing the uterus for a pregnancy by securing a sufficient blood supply and by preventing the uterus from contracting and losing a fertilized egg.

Sperm can fertilize the ready egg in the fallopian tube during a 6 to 12 hour period. Fertilization happens when a sperm enters the egg and the embryo starts to form. Two cells divide and become four, the four cells divide and become eight, and so on. By the time the cluster of cells reaches the uterus and settles down into the lining of the uterus, it has become an embryo.

This settling down is called implantation. It takes about seven days from fertilization to implantation. The rise of estrogen and progesterone in the blood stream of the woman, along with the pregnancy hormone HCG from cells surrounding the embryo, signals pregnancy. From now on, the female body concentrates on the growth of the embryo and stops the cycle until a few weeks after the baby is born. This is why women cannot conceive again while they are pregnant. A woman can only have one pregnancy at a time, but this does not exclude the possibility of having more than one embryo or fetus at a time, e.g. twins.

The rise in estrogen and progesterone signals to the ovaries: Do not produce any more eggs for now. We have to take care of this embryo first! A pregnancy test can be positive 8-10 days after ovulation. If no fertilization of the egg occurs, the production of progesterone stops. So does the production of estrogens. The message is basically: We do not have a fertilized egg to produce an embryo this month, so stop all the preparations and start all over again! The end of the story is that the thickened lining of the uterus, which was supposed to be the bed for the fertilized egg, is no longer necessary. The same applies to the egg, which did not get fertilized. The body rids itself of this bedding and the egg by bleeding. This is known as the period or menstruation.

## The link to contraception

This was a brief description of what's happening with our bodies when it comes to reproduction. What does this have to do with contraception then? Remember we were talking about the principles of contraception:

- Hormonal methods: make the body believe that the ovaries produce hormones while they are, in fact, resting and not producing eggs. Most hormonal methods stop ovulation.
- Barrier methods: prevent sperm and egg from meeting each other.
- Chemical methods (spermicides): destroy sperm upon contact.
- Surgical methods: interrupt the transportation route of eggs or sperm.
- Emergency contraception: delays egg release.

**In 2000, the fertility rate for adolescents (number of pregnancies per 1,000 women of reproductive age) was 17.3 compared with 33.9 for women in the 35-39 age group and 5.9 for women in the 40-44 age group.**

**The highest abortion rates (number of abortions per 1,000 women) occur in women 18-19 years and 20-24 years of age.**

Did you know that a woman could become pregnant even...
- When she has intercourse for the first time?
- When she has her period?
- If she had no period yet?
- If her partner ejaculates not inside her vagina but close by?

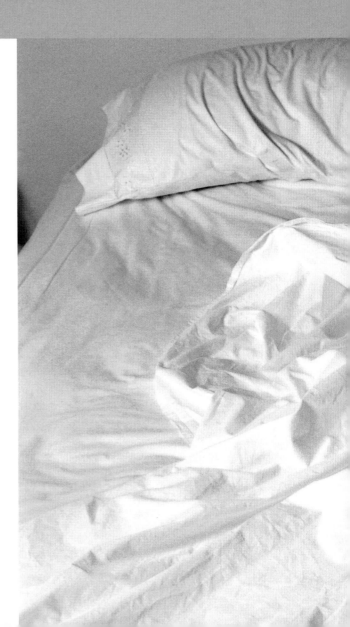

Blood could come from wounds in your mouth, on your lips, or anywhere on your body, from menstrual periods, from injecting needles, or from piercing and tattoo needles.

Body fluids are semen, sperm, pre-ejaculatory fluid (fluid, which comes out of the penis during sexual arousal), saliva, breast milk, and vaginal fluids.

## The decisions you make

Your risk of getting an STI will be higher if you...

- have unprotected oral, vaginal, or anal sex with someone you are not 100% sure does not have an STI (see safer sex section later in this chapter for more details)
- have sex under the influence of alcohol or drugs
- or your partner share or have shared sex toys without taking the proper precautions (cleansing of toys and condom use)
- or your partner have shared needles or equipment for drugs, steroids, body piercing, or tattoos
- or your partner have shared toothbrushes or razors
- or your partner have had sex with other people prior to or during your current relationship

You are also at higher risk if...

- your partner has an STI, or has had an STI in the past
- you have a new sex partner, or have had more than 2 partners in the past 6 months

## Risky facts

Statistically, certain groups of people are at higher risk of contracting STIs. Often, this is because of higher-risk behaviours associated with that group, such as higher rates of unprotected sex and/or a tendency to have more sexual partners. Your risk is also increased because of the larger number of infected people in the group, making it more likely that you will be exposed to an infected person.

These groups include...

- persons emigrating from countries with high rates of STIs
- commercial sex workers, including those who have "survival sex" (exchanging sex for money, drugs, shelter or food)
- men who have sex with men (MSM)
- youth under age 25; STIs are most common in young adults under the age of 25; women in the age group 15-19 have the highest rate of STIs in Canada.

STI (sexually transmitted infection) and STD (sexually transmitted disease) are two terms for the same thing. The more precise term is STI (plural: STIs), the term we use throughout this book. The infection comes first and it is the infection which needs to be prevented. A disease process only starts after an infection.

## PARASITIC AND FUNGAL SEXUALLY TRANSMITTED INFECTIONS

| Name of STI | How you get it | How long before you may notice symptoms? | What if you are pregnant? | How are you treated? | How are you tested? | Other comments |
|---|---|---|---|---|---|---|
| Trichomoniasis | Unprotected vaginal intercourse. Contact with infested towels, clothes, bedding and washcloths. | 4 to 28 days with symptoms taking up to 6 months to appear in some. | Your baby may be born with a low weight or prematurely. | Curable with oral medication. | Health care provider will examine you and possibly take a sample from your vagina. | May contribute to development of Pelvic Inflammatory Disease and infertility.<br><br>Often no symptoms in men, but can be present in the urethra. |
| Pubic Lice / Crabs and Scabies | Close contact, sexual and non-sexual. Contact with infested bed sheets, towels and clothes. Not from pets. | Symptoms occur when they bite or burrow into your skin. | Medications to treat them can be harmful to an unborn baby, so check with your health care provider or pharmacist first. | Creams, lotions or shampoos are used to get rid of them. | Health care provider will look at your skin and hair. | Usually in pubic hair, but may also be found on chest, armpit, eyelash and facial hair.<br><br>Wash clothes and bed linen in hot water, or dry-clean and press with a very hot iron. Freezing clothes, fabrics or blankets or storing them in an air-tight plastic bag for two weeks will also destroy the insects and their eggs. |
| Candidiasis / Yeast Infection | Generally not sexually transmitted. It is related to the presence of other infections and health of the vagina. It can also be related to your general health. Men can get an infection on their penis from vaginal sex. | Varies according to vaginal and general health. | Often present in pregnancy; does not harm the baby. The baby can develop an oral infection during birth. | Pills, creams or ointments. Talk to your doctor if it is your first infection. | Health care provider will examine you and possibly take a sample from your vagina. | It is often considered an STI because it is seen in women with other types of vaginal and reproductive infections.<br><br>A majority of women will experience a yeast infection at least once in their lives. |

## Human Papillomavirus (HPV) and Cancer

There are many different types of HPV, some which cause symptoms such as visible warts (growths) and others which cause changes in your cells that can become cancerous. The types of HPV that cause genital warts (visible) are not linked to cancer. But, because you could have more than one type of HPV you could be at risk for both warts and cancer.

HPV and the changes that can occur in the cells are typically on the cervix in women. It takes years for cervical cancer to develop, upwards of 20, in those with HPV types that are linked to cancer (called high risk types), but precancerous changes can occur within a couple of years. There are often no symptoms associated with precancerous or cancerous changes in the cervix. Therefore, it is important to test for these changes. Testing for HPV cannot tell you if you have changes in your cells. This is done by testing the cells specifically through a Pap smear. Testing for HPV can be used in conjunction with the Pap to provide more information to the health care provider.

There have also been links of HPV to anal, penile and vulvar cancers, therefore regular medical check ups are an important part of your health.

# VIRAL SEXUALLY TRANSMITTED INFECTIONS

| Name of STI | How you get it | How long before you may notice symptoms? | Effects on baby during pregnancy and at birth | How you are tested and treated | Other comments |
|---|---|---|---|---|---|
| Genital Herpes | Direct contact with sores or intact/ healthy looking skin in the genital and anal region of an infected individual. Unprotected vaginal, oral or anal sex with an infected partner. Contact with cold sores (on the mouth) to the genitals can cause genital herpes. | In 2 to 21 days. A large number of people do not notice symptoms. | The baby can be infected during pregnancy or at birth, resulting in lesions to the skin and/or serious infection, which can lead to death. | A swab may be taken of any sores. You may need to give a blood sample. No cure exists. There are treatments to decrease symptoms or suppress recurrent outbreaks. | If you touch herpes sores, wash your hands with soap and water to avoid spreading the infection. Prior to an outbreak, a person may feel a tingling or burning sensation in the spot where the virus first entered the skin. Sores can also be internal (cervical, urethral, oral or rectal). |
| Human Papillomavirus (HPV)/Genital Warts | Contact during sex, vaginal, anal or oral with infected area of the body, which can be internal or external. Direct contact, skin to skin, with an infected person. | 1 to 8 months for visible warts, but a lot of people do not have any visible/noticeable symptoms. | The baby can be infected during birth. | Typically a physical exam to locate visible warts. No treatment to cure it. Can treat the visible warts, which may also go away on their own in some people. Symptoms can return after treatment. Typically treated by freezing, burning, or using creams or other medications applied to the skin. | Link to cervical cancer (see page 18 for explanation and related testing). They grow in moist areas such as the penis, the vagina, the cervix, the anus, the scrotum and the thighs. Warts may appear on the lips or in the mouth after oral sex with an infected person, but this is not common. |
| Hepatitis B | Unprotected anal, vaginal or oral sex. Contact with blood, both sexual and non sexual contact (e.g. sharing toothbrush, razor). | In 2 to 6 months | The baby can be infected during pregnancy or at birth. | You can be tested by a blood sample. Most adults can clear the infection on their own, after which they are likely immune; others become lifetime carriers, can develop liver damage and can pass it on. There is treatment to help decrease the effects of the virus on the liver. | There is a vaccine to prevent it, ask your health care provider. Having HIV at the same time can result in greater/faster damage to the liver. |
| Hepatitis A | Unprotected oral-anal contact. Ingestion of feces from unclean hands, food, water and utensils. | In 15 to 50 days | Typically no effect on baby. | Usually no treatment is necessary, it clears in 2 to 6 months, and then you are typically immune. Some people may require hospitalization if symptoms are severe. You can be tested by a blood sample. | High rate of fatal complications when co-infected with other hepatitis viruses (e.g. Hepatitis C which is caught through blood, primarily by sharing needles and drug equipment) or HIV. There is a vaccine to prevent it. Ask your health care provider. |
| HIV/Human Immunodeficiency Virus | Contact with body fluids such as blood, semen, pre-semen, vaginal fluids, and breast milk, which must enter your body. Not transmitted through casual contact (shaking hands, hugging). Not transmitted by sneezing or coughing. Not transmitted through insects or animals. The HIV virus can also be found in saliva (spit), sweat and tears, but only in very low amounts. These body fluids are not known to spread HIV infection. | From months to years, varies between people. | The baby can be infected during pregnancy, at birth or through breast feeding. | A blood test can tell if you have HIV. It is called the HIV antibody test. HIV has what they call a 3-month window period (for most people), which is the time it takes your body to develop the antibodies that they test for. Your test will therefore not tell you if you have been infected by any sexual activity that occurred in the 3 months prior to the test. This can be up to 6 months in some individuals, depending on your health. Ask about anonymous HIV testing. No cure. Treatment for symptoms and to slow down progression to AIDS. | Attacks your immune system. Progresses to AIDS when your immune system is damaged and you get other infections and cancers. A person can be re-infected with the HIV virus more than once, affecting progression and treatment. If you are HIV positive and have another of the sexually transmitted infections, you increase your chances of giving HIV to your partner. If you don't have HIV but have another sexually transmitted infection, you increase your chances of getting HIV from an HIV positive partner. |

# BACTERIAL SEXUALLY TRANSMITTED INFECTIONS

| Name of STI | How you get it | How long before you may notice symptoms | Where you may notice symptoms | What if you are pregnant? | Long term effects of repeat and untreated infections | How are you tested? | How are you treated? |
|---|---|---|---|---|---|---|---|
| Chlamydia | Unprotected oral, vaginal and anal sex. | 2 to 6 weeks. Most do not have symptoms. | Eyes, throat, rectum, vagina and urethra. | Baby can develop pneumonia or eye infections during birth. | Pelvic Inflammatory Disease (PID, see below), infertility, and ectopic pregnancy (see glossary) for women. Inflammation of the testes and epididymitis in men, which may affect fertility. | Urine or swab from the infected area. | Curable with antibiotics. |
| Gonorrhea | Unprotected oral, vaginal and anal sex. | 2 to 7 days. Most do not have symptoms. | Throat, rectum, vagina and urethra. | Baby can develop eye infections during birth. | PID, infertility and ectopic pregnancy in women. Inflammation of the testes and epididymitis in men, which may affect fertility. | Swab from the infected area. Urine testing is available in some areas. | Curable with antibiotics. |
| Syphilis | Unprotected oral, vaginal and anal sex. Rarely through contact with blood. Can transmit it during primary, secondary and early latent phase (less than a year). | Symptoms appear in stages: primary, secondary, latent and tertiary. Symptoms of earlier stages appear from days to months after exposure. Late latent and tertiary can take up to and beyond 30 years. | Mouth, genital and anal region; as it progresses to later stages, symptoms can be found throughout the body, e.g. rash on feet and hands. | Baby can be infected during pregnancy during primary, secondary and latent stage, possibly leading to birth defects and death. Baby can also be infected at birth. | With tertiary stage irreversible damage to internal organs, such as heart and brain. | Swab of any sores and/or blood sample. | Curable with antibiotics, length varies with stage of infection. Damage from late stages is not reversed with treatment. |
| Lyphogranuloma Venereum / LGV | Unprotected oral, vaginal and anal sex. | 3 days to 2 months. Symptoms progress in stages: primary, secondary and tertiary. | Throat, rectum, vagina, urethra and glands in the infected area. | Baby can be infected during birth. | Swelling and damage to glands in the groin and neck. Scarring and irreversible damage to genitals and rectum. | Swab of any sores, blood sample or fluid sample from swollen glands. | Curable with antibiotics. Damage from tertiary stage is not reversed with typical treatment, may require surgery. |

**PID:** Pelvic inflammatory disease is the result of an infection moving up the female reproductive tract (uterus and fallopian tubes) causing swelling and scarring. This can lead to chronic pelvic pain, infertility, or ectopic pregnancy. Antibiotics will be given to take for a couple of weeks. Follow up with a health care provider is important as treatment may not be effective in some cases. Hospitalization may be required.

**Chlamydia:** The number of people infected has been increasing since 1997. Those between 15 and 24 years of age are most at risk of contracting this infection and make up over two-thirds of nationally reported cases.

## Impact of STIs on women

A consequence of untreated STIs can be infertility. It seems unfair, but women suffer more severe long-term consequences including infertility, pelvic inflammatory disease, ectopic pregnancy, chronic pelvic pain and cervical cancer. Women are also less likely to see a doctor if they are infected because many STIs in women have no symptoms and the infection is more difficult to diagnose.

## No symptoms — no worries: not quite!

Preventing STIs isn't always easy. One of the biggest problems is that MOST PEOPLE WHO GET AN STI HAVE NO VISIBLE OR NOTICABLE SYMPTOMS, AND THEREFORE MAY NOT REALIZE THEY ARE INFECTED. If you do have symptoms they can include...

- different or heavier discharge from the vagina
- inflamed, sore and itchy vagina
- vaginal odour
- vaginal bleeding between periods or after intercourse
- discharge from the penis
- pain or swelling in the penis, testicles, scrotum
- discharge or pain from the anus
- a burning feeling when urinating (peeing)
- sores in the genital region, the anal region or the mouth
- appearance of a rash anywhere on the body
- swollen glands in the groin
- pain in the lower abdomen
- fever and chills
- itching, tingling and irritation of the genital and anal region
- sore throat
- joint pain
- pain during sex
- growths on or around the genitals or anal area
- redness, swelling and discharge from your eye
- poor appetite, nausea and vomiting
- headaches, feeling very tired
- jaundice (yellow colouring of the eyes and skin)
- dark coloured urine, pale colored stool

This list covers most of the common symptoms for STIs; but STIs may cause other symptoms or none at all. Having one or more of these symptoms doesn't necessarily mean you have an STI, but if you are having these symptoms you should see a health care provider for testing.

Remember symptoms can appear days, weeks, months or even years after you have been exposed to an STI. So, even if you don't have any symptoms, it doesn't mean you don't have an STI – the only way to know for sure is to get tested.

If you are not having any symptoms but are at higher risk because of your behaviour, you may also want to see your health care provider for testing.

## To be sure: TESTING

Once an infection enters your body, it begins to cause changes in your body. This takes time. Symptoms won't appear right away, if they appear at all. If a person is tested too soon after they became infected, there's a chance the test will not detect the STI or the changes it causes. The time period between infection and when a test will detect that infection is different for each STI. For example, HIV testing requires a three month window period, the usual amount of time it takes for your body to react to the virus. Testing before three months has passed may not detect the infection even if the person is HIV positive. For this reason, it's important to ask your health care provider when is an appropriate time to test.

## If you test positive

If you test positive for an STI, it is important to notify your sexual partner(s) immediately so they can also be treated, and to prevent them from passing the infection on to someone else or back to you. Your health care provider or a public health professional may notify your partner(s) for you. You can discuss these options with your health care provider.

If you do test positive for an STI it is important to follow all your health care provider's exact instructions. In particular you should...

- make sure you take your medication until it is completely finished, even if your symptoms have disappeared
- go to your health care provider for a follow-up appointment if advised to do so
- ask your health care provider how soon after treatment you can have sexual intercourse
- if you are pregnant, make sure that treatments and medication are safe for you and the baby

Remember:

- Health care providers are not mind readers. If you don't tell them what you're feeling or what kinds of things you've been doing, they won't be able to fully help you.
- You can catch some STIs more than once, and you can have more than one STI at the same time.
- Just because you have recently tested negative or have taken all your medication doesn't mean you are protected, you may still be at risk depending on your behaviour.

## Safer sex

There won't always be clues that someone has an STI, so insist on safer sex even if your partner says he or she is "safe". And by the way: What does "safe" or "free of STI/HIV" mean? **Each partner in a monogamous relationship should have two negative HIV antibody tests at least six months apart and each partner should have other appropriate STI tests performed with negative results.**

People can't always tell if they have an STI – without proper testing, you can't tell for sure if you're infected. Neither can your partner.

So what do we mean when we talk about unprotected sex?

## Unprotected sex

Unprotected sex means that there is no barrier between you and your partner's body fluids (vaginal fluids, semen/pre-cum, blood) or between you and your partner's urethra, anus, mouth or vagina. This typically means not using a condom or using one improperly, such as putting on the condom after sex has already started or taking it off before you're finished. A condom can also break or slip off during sex. Condoms are only dependable if you use them. If you only use them sometimes, you're still at risk. It only takes one unprotected sexual encounter to transfer an STI.

The only 100% safe sex is abstinence from all sexual activity, or sex within a completely mutually monogamous relationship: you only have sex with one person and he/she only has sex with you – in which both partners are STI-free.

Keep in mind that activities other than just sexual intercourse can transmit STIs – sharing infected needles, sex toys, razors, toothbrushes, etc. – so it's important to consider these activities too. Talk to your partner and define your expectations and limits.

A lot of people feel that they don't have to worry about STIs if they're in a monogamous relationship, but you may still be at risk. Many people have what are called "serial" monogamous relationships: a series of faithful, mutually monogamous relationships, **one after the other.** These relationships are often

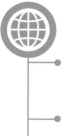

**The 2004 Global Sex Survey revealed that among Canadian participants:**

42% had unprotected sex within the last 12 months without knowing their partner's sexual history, although the top concerns when it comes to sex were:

HIV/AIDS: 54%

Unplanned pregnancy: 30%

with "known and trusted" partners, but because STIs vary in terms of the amount of time it takes to detect them or develop symptoms if they appear at all, there may still be risk involved. You and your partners should get tested!

Some STIs may never show symptoms and others may take years, so without testing there is no way to be 100 percent sure. Again, keep in mind that testing may not be accurate if you've recently had sex outside of the relationship. If you are waiting to be tested, or waiting for your results, continue to use protection until you know for sure. Make sure you tell your partner what you expect from them in a monogamous relationship since people's definitions may vary. Don't assume because you are not having sex outside the relationship that they are not.

### Protected sex with condoms

When used correctly, a condom provides a barrier between your body fluids and your partner's, and can help protect against both STIs and pregnancy.

- Use a condom for oral, vaginal and anal sex, or when sharing sex toys. Use a condom when performing oral sex on a man. For a woman, place a condom cut length-wise or dental dam over the contact area. This can also be used for rimming (oral/anal contact).
- The male condom covers the penis. A female condom is a liner worn in the vagina. Although there have been reports of the female condom being used in the rectum for anal sex, this is not a recommended use by manufacturers. Used anally, current research has noted slippage, discomfort and an increase in rectal bleeding. Remember to not use the male and female condom together.
- Practice before you need it. This is especially true of the female condom.
- Latex is the most common material in condoms, but synthetic (polyurethane) male and female condoms also offer protection. These are particularly useful for people sensitive or allergic to latex.
- Oil-based products (like petroleum jelly, vaginal cream) can weaken a latex condom and should be avoided.

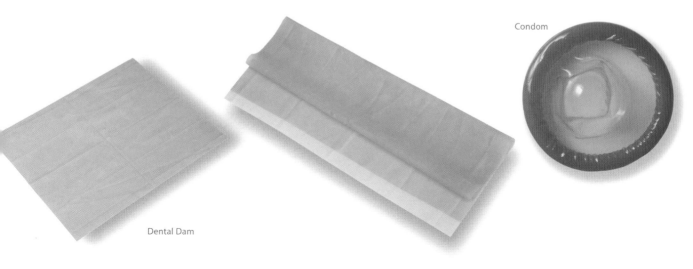

Condom

Dental Dam

**FREQUENTLY ASKED QUESTIONS**

**?**  **Can I get infected the first time I have sex?**

Yes.

**?**  **Can I get infected even without "real" intercourse (the guy ejaculates outside the vagina, also referred to as outercourse)?**

Yes.

**?**  **Will my parents find out about the STI testing?**

No. Your doctor or any health care provider has to ensure your privacy even if you are under age.

**?**  **Do I have to tell my partner if I am infected?**

Yes, you should. Your partner (or your recent partners, if you have had more than one) has to know about your infection so that he/she can go for testing and treatment as well.

**?**  **What to do when the test is positive?**

Depending on the kind of STI you have, your doctor will prescribe treatment and will tell you how to protect yourself and your partner during treatment. Also refer to the phone numbers in the reference section of this book.

**?**  **Will I get cured?**

You will have to discuss the infection and the treatment with your doctor. Generally speaking, bacterial infections can be cured with antibiotics, especially when they are detected early. Viral infections can be treated but not cured. For example, medication taken for herpes helps to decrease your symptoms. This does not mean that you are cured and therefore you may still pass it on to your partners.

**?**  **Is there a sex life after I've been cured from an STI?**

Of course! But you might use this experience to protect yourself in the future and practice safer sex! And...there is no excuse because this book tells you how...do it!

**?**  **Are vaccinations available?**

Not at this time. The only vaccination available is one for hepatitis B. If you get an STI once, you can always get it again.

**?**  **Is it possible to have more than one STI at a time?**

Yes. Keep in mind: many STIs are easily treated, but all can be dangerous if ignored.

**Define your own boundaries, know your limits. What amount of risk are you willing to take?**
**What steps are you willing and able to take to protect yourself and your partner from STIs?**
**If you don't use protection, ask yourself "why not?" Or why don't you use it consistently?**

- Natural membrane condoms (also called "sheepskin" condoms) do not offer the same degree of protection against some viral STIs, including HIV and hepatitis.
- Nonoxynol-9 spermicide is a chemical that may cause irritation and increase the risk of HIV transmission. Use condoms without nonoxynol-9.
- Check the expiry date ("Exp.") on the condom packaging. If you can't find the expiry date or the date has passed, don't use the condom.
- If the condom has been exposed to extreme temperatures don't use it.
- Although condoms provide protection against most STIs, a condom is not 100% safe. A condom has its disadvantages. It does not cover the whole genital area of both partners, meaning that you may not be protected from STIs, which can be transmitted by skin-to-skin contact. These STIs include human papillomavirus (HPV) and herpes.
- In fact, except for abstinence, there are no 100% effective ways to prevent STIs, which are transmitted by skin-to-skin contact. Condoms will reduce the risk, but if the condom does not separate your body from an infected area or fluid, it may not prevent transmission.

### Some more tips

- Performing oral sex should be avoided immediately after brushing your teeth, after using dental floss, or if either partner has sores or cuts in the mouth. It should also be avoided if either partner has recently had any kind of dental or invasive procedure in the mouth.
- Masturbation alone is safe. If masturbating with others, make sure to avoid any contact/exchange of blood or body fluids, especially if there are any openings in the skin.

**IN SUMMARY:**
Anyone who is involved in any sexual activity, including intercourse, can get infected with an STI. Safer sex reduces this risk. The good news: most STIs can be cured; others can be controlled. The bad news: some, such as HIV, can even kill you.

Protect yourself and your partner by practicing safer sex.

No condom?   No sex.   or:   No glove? No love.

This chapter is about hormonal methods of contraception.
There are seven methods to choose from:

**Oral contraceptive pill**
(contains estrogen and progestin)

**Transdermal contraceptive patch**
(contains estrogen and progestin)

**Contraceptive ring**
(contains estrogen and progestin)

**Progestin-only pill**
(contains only progestin)

**Injectable contraceptive**
(contains only progestin)

**Implant**
(contains only progestin)

**Intrauterine system (IUS)**
(contains only progestin) refer to chapter 7

# REMOTE CONTROL

## THE PILL AND OTHER HORMONAL METHODS

The comparison chart on pages 28-29 will give you a brief overview of these methods.

Hormones are substances in the body that convey messages from one organ to another. For a refresher course on hormones visit the basics in Chapter 1. We can compare hormonal contraception to the remote control of a TV. The press of a certain button leads to a reaction in your TV. Hormonal methods work with hormones as "buttons" or couriers, which make certain changes to your system and very effectively prevent the woman from becoming pregnant. This comparison should not, however, make you believe that you can switch these methods on or off like a TV! It takes a while for the body to adjust to the hormones. Going on and off the pill for example would unnecessarily put you at risk of becoming pregnant.

Here are the features of this group of methods. They...
- are the most effective reversible contraceptives apart from the IUD and the IUS
- require minimal effort and skills in order to be used correctly
- are independent of intercourse
- offer many health benefits apart from reliable contraception
- do not protect against STIs and HIV
- are designed for long-term use
- make changes to the system of your body and may have unwanted effects which normally disappear after the first 1-3 months of use
- efficacy of hormonal methods may be reduced in overweight users

Hormonal methods are the most popular contraceptives in Canada. In the 2002 Canadian Contraception Study, 34% of respondents were using hormonal methods.

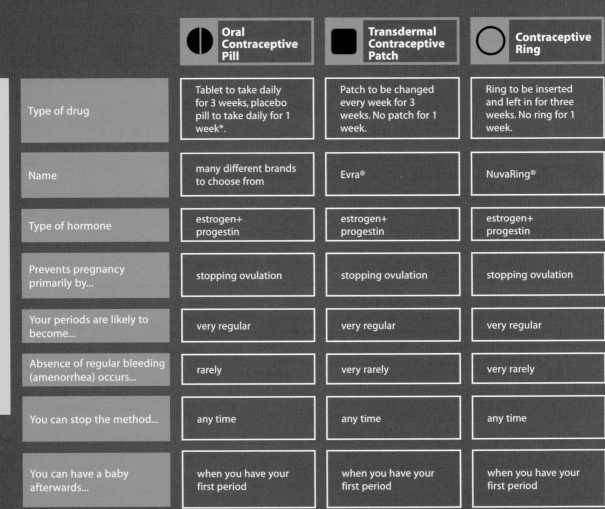

**COMPARE AND DECIDE:**
Hormonal Methods of Contraception

| | Oral Contraceptive Pill | Transdermal Contraceptive Patch | Contraceptive Ring |
|---|---|---|---|
| Type of drug | Tablet to take daily for 3 weeks, placebo pill to take daily for 1 week*. | Patch to be changed every week for 3 weeks. No patch for 1 week. | Ring to be inserted and left in for three weeks. No ring for 1 week. |
| Name | many different brands to choose from | Evra® | NuvaRing® |
| Type of hormone | estrogen+ progestin | estrogen+ progestin | estrogen+ progestin |
| Prevents pregnancy primarily by... | stopping ovulation | stopping ovulation | stopping ovulation |
| Your periods are likely to become... | very regular | very regular | very regular |
| Absence of regular bleeding (amenorrhea) occurs... | rarely | very rarely | very rarely |
| You can stop the method... | any time | any time | any time |
| You can have a baby afterwards... | when you have your first period | when you have your first period | when you have your first period |

*1 week of placebo pills are only supplied in 28-day packs. They are also referred to as "sugar pills".

| POP Progestin-only Pill | Injectable Contraceptive | Implant | IUS (see chapter 7) |
|---|---|---|---|
| Tablet to take every day. No breaks. | Injection in muscle of upper arm, buttocks or thigh every 10-13 weeks. No interruptions. | Implant under skin of upper arm every 3-5 years. | One insertion every 5 years. |
| Micronor® | Depo-Provera® | Norplant® Implanon® | Mirena® |
| progestin only | progestin only | progestin only | progestin only |
| changing lining of uterus, thickening mucus | stopping ovulation | changing lining of uterus, thickening mucus | changing lining of uterus |
| somewhat irregular | sparse | somewhat irregular | sparse |
| occasionally | very often | often | often |
| any time | only after the 12-week interval is over | any time (appointment for removal necessary) | any time |
| when you have your first period | when you have your first period (up to 9 months after the last injection) | when you have your first period | when you have your first period |

# ORAL CONTRACEPTIVE PILL

### Who controls the show?
The woman.

### What is the pill all about?
The pill has to be taken daily whether you have sex or not. It contains two types of hormones (estrogen and progestin).

The pill replaces the natural female cycle by an artificial one. The ovaries temporarily stop their hormone production and there is no ovulation thus making pregnancy almost impossible. The pill also changes the mucus in the cervix and the lining of the uterus. This "triple action" makes the pill extremely effective in preventing pregnancy.

### How do I get it?
See a family physician, a gynaecologist, a school nurse or a family planning clinic. A physical exam is recommended but not always necessary and not always performed.

### How effective is the pill in preventing unintended pregnancy?
92-99.7% effective.

### Does it protect against sexually transmitted infections and HIV?
No.

### What makes this method so special?
- It is a highly effective, reversible method of contraception.
- It offers additional health benefits such as more regular cycles, reduced menstrual flow, improvement of acne, and it protects against certain cancers.
- It is the most researched method.

### Possible problems
There might be some unwanted effects such as irregular bleeding, breast tenderness, headaches, and nausea. They usually disappear after the first few cycles.

### Necessary routine
Take pill daily.

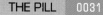

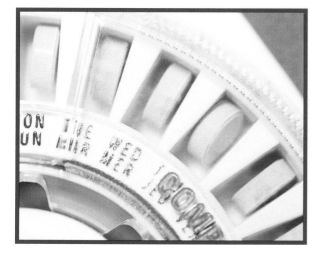

## WHAT IS THE PILL ALL ABOUT?

The oral contraceptive pill (OC) or simply "the pill" is one of the most researched and at the same time the most misunderstood drug in the world.

About 100 million women all over the world are relying on it and it is one of the most prescribed medications. The pill may be suitable for any healthy woman, regardless of age. It should not be used for a month at a time but should be used for several months (or even several years) in a row. Some people only want to take the pill when they are in a stable relationship and they stop taking it when the relationship ends. This is not a good idea. It puts you at risk of unintended pregnancy if you have intercourse before you have started to use a contraceptive method again.

There are also many myths and misconceptions surrounding the pill. Please refer to page 32 to get an idea about false impressions. You may even believe some of them yourself but let us give you a better picture!

# MYTH

# FACT

**MYTHS AND MISCONCEPTIONS**

| | |
|---|---|
| The pill causes cancer | WRONG. In fact, the pill reduces the risk for certain cancers. |
| The pill can cause acne | WRONG. In fact, some OCs even reduce acne. |
| Women who take the pill should have periodic pill breaks | WRONG. In fact, the pill puts your ovaries to rest. Once your system is used to the pill you should keep on taking it to avoid irregular cycles and to keep the protection against pregnancy. Also, side effects of the pill do not increase with time. |
| The pill delays future fertility | WRONG. In fact, most women can get pregnant immediately after stopping the pill. It is a good idea, though, to wait until you have had at least one normal period before trying to become pregnant. |
| All women aged 35 and over must stop taking the pill | WRONG. A healthy, non-smoking woman can take the pill until menopause. You have to stop the pill at age 35 only if you are a smoker or have other health problems. |
| The pill causes weight gain | WRONG. Weight gain is normally due to an increased appetite and lack of exercise. Just as many women lose weight while taking the pill as gain weight. Studies could not confirm any relationship between the use of the pill and weight gain. Although the estrogen in the OC may sometimes cause a woman to feel bloated in the beginning, this feeling normally improves with time. |
| It is more risky to take the pill than to be pregnant | WRONG. In fact, the risks of taking the pill have been thoroughly studied and are lower than the risks of pregnancy. |
| The pill causes birth defects if you become pregnant while taking the pill | WRONG. In fact, studies and many years of observation have confirmed that the pill does not cause birth defects if taken when a pregnancy has begun. |

Many people do not know that the pill offers many health benefits in addition to reliable contraception. Have a look at the circle graphic on page 35. We will give you a complete picture of the pill for you to judge, together with your physician, whether this method is the right choice for you. We want you to be comfortable with your choice. If you have any problems, questions or concerns discuss them with your health care provider. These people are there for you.

## How does the pill work?

Oral contraceptives contain two different hormones, a progestin and an estrogen. These hormones, which are similar to the ones produced in your own body, tell the ovaries not to let any egg cells ripen. In a way, the ovaries are put to sleep.

During OC use the lining of the uterus becomes thinner and the entrance to the uterus is blocked by a thicker mucus, which makes it more difficult for sperm to move and to reach the uterus. This is called the "triple action of the pill", which makes it such an effective method of contraception.

In the 7-day hormone-free interval, bleeding starts just like in the normal cycle but it is usually less heavy than in women who do not take the pill. Some women don't even bleed, which is ok. Since the pill actually replaces the normal cycle we do not call this a normal menstruation or period but "withdrawal bleeding", which is caused by the withdrawal of estrogen in the hormone-free interval.

## How effective is the pill in preventing unintended pregnancy?

The pill is 99.7% effective when used perfectly, making it a very reliable reversible method of contraception. There is a "user failure rate" of 8%. It is a statistic that reflects that some women make mistakes in taking the pill or that there are certain interactions with other drugs taken at the same time. The pill is as effective as the POP, the ring, and the patch. A little joke on the side: Do you know what the most effective oral contraceptive of them all is? The word NO!

## Does the pill protect against sexually transmitted infections and HIV?

No. The pill does not protect against sexually transmitted infections and HIV. The simple recipe for safer sex is dual protection! Use a condom (male condom or female condom) for protection against STIs and HIV and take the pill for protection against pregnancy!

## How popular is the pill in Canada?

In the 2002 Canadian Contraception Study, the pill was used by 32% of women. It is the most popular method of contraception in Canada, the method women are most familiar with and have the most favourable opinion of.

## The pill may be a good choice for you if you are looking for a method that...

- is simple and very effective
- makes periods more regular, with less bleeding and less pain
- you can use from teenage years to menopause
- allows spontaneity
- allows you to become pregnant when you stop taking it
- offers you additional health benefits, known as non-contraceptive benefits

Look at the statistics below to get an idea why Canadian women started taking the pill.

| The 2002 Canadian Contraception Study revealed the following main reasons why women chose to take the pill... | |
| --- | --- |
| **71%** | wanted a contraceptive |
| **31%** | wanted relief from irregular periods |
| **27%** | wanted relief from painful periods |

## The pill is not for you, if...
- you have problems with taking a pill every day, even if you do not have sex
- you are planning to take it on and off depending on the state of a sexual relationship
- you have certain health problems that you have to discuss with your doctor (see list below)

## Where do I get the pill?
You should make an appointment with a family physician, a gynaecologist, a public health clinic, or a family planning clinic. You can also contact the health service in your school. Some health services provide you with the pill without a prescription. You will be asked to go for a check-up to obtain the prescription later. Please consider the following:

- **You're not too crazy about going to a physician for a health exam?**
  Then you might have the idea of borrowing pills from your best girlfriend. Do not even think of it! Your girlfriend's pills were prescribed for her and they might not be good for you!

- **You are afraid that your parents might find out.**
  If you do not want your parents to know that you are taking the pill, you should ask your doctor to keep it secret. The doctor does not need to talk to your parents and he/she will not ask permission from your parents to prescribe the pill for you. This is not necessary in Canada. We believe that you are old enough to make responsible decisions about your health.

- **You are afraid of the exam - the pelvic exam?**
  Do not worry - it is not a big deal. A pelvic exam is not always necessary. With this exam your doctor wants to make sure that your reproductive organs are healthy.

## What to expect on your visit
The first part of your visit will consist of questions the doctor will ask you about your health and lifestyle, any previous diseases you may have had, medications you are taking and about your family's health. Some questions might seem a bit too intimate but keep in mind that the physician is on your side.

(Continued on page 38)

# FOR SOME WOMEN THE PILL MAY NOT BE THE RIGHT CHOICE IF...

→ You are pregnant

→ You have or have had blood clots in your legs or elsewhere in your body

→ You have high blood pressure

→ You suffer from migraine headaches with aura

→ You have cancer of the breast or other sex organs, or there is a suspicion of a cancer

→ You have had a stroke or heart attack

→ You have a liver tumour or severe liver disease

→ You are a smoker and are over 35 years of age

→ You delivered a baby less than 6 weeks ago and are breastfeeding

→ You have diabetes with end-organ involvement

**Women who take
the pill have:**

- more regular cycles

- less painful periods and fewer symptoms around the time of their periods

- increased bone mineral density

- decreased excess of facial and body hair (hirsutism)

- a 50% lower risk of ovarian cancer after five years of taking the pill

- a 50% lower risk of endometrial cancer

- possibly fewer benign ovarian cysts and breast diseases

- fewer bleeding irregularities and hot flushes when starting menopause

- lower risk of inflammation of the fallopian tubes, which can lead to infertility and chronic pelvic pain

- lose less blood during menstruation and have a lower risk of iron deficiency anemia

- suffer less from acne

**And the great thing about it:
some of these protective effects
even continue for years after you
stop taking the pill.**

NON-CONTRACEPTIVE BENEFITS OF ORAL CONTRACEPTIVES

**HOW DO I GET STARTED?**

**Start while you are having your menses (the first 5 days of your menstrual cycle)**

**1** Study the package insert. It sounds like a boring idea but...the package inserts of OCs are well done. They tell you a great deal about the pill you chose.

**2** Make use of the stickers and other support tools to help you remember to take the pill regularly.

**3** Call your doctor immediately if certain problems occur. Like any other medication, side effects can occur which need immediate attention. In your package insert you can read about these warning signs.

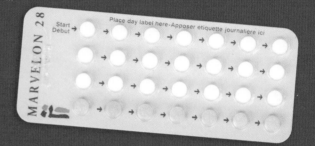

**How do I get the routine, how to remember?**

When you start taking the pill during the first five days of your cycle you enjoy protection against pregnancy immediately. The first tablet in every pack that follows will always be taken on the same day of the week.

If you start taking the pill on a later day in the cycle you have to use a backup method of contraception for the first 21 days. Some health care providers may encourage you to take your first pill while you are in their office ("Quick Start"). If you are not within the first five days of your cycle you need to use a backup method.

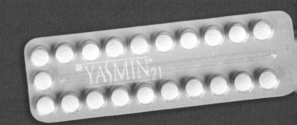

There are tools to remember to take the pill everyday, such as electronic cards, e-mail, text message reminders, etc. Contact your physician, pharmacist or the manufacturer of your OC brand to obtain one of these handy tools.

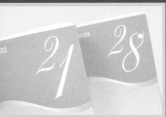

### Here is how to take the pill:

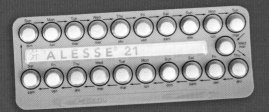

**Monophasic 21-day pack:**
In a 21-day pack **all pills contain hormones.** Take the first pill of the pack during the first 5 days of your cycle. Take one pill every day until the pack is finished. Then wait seven days and start the next pack. During the seven-day hormone-free interval you will probably experience bleeding. However, it is very important that you start your new pack after seven days regardless of whether bleeding has occurred or not, or whether it is still going on.

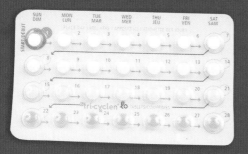

**Monophasic 28-day pack:**
In a 28-day pack only the first 21 pills contain hormones. Different colours indicate the two types of pills (hormonal pills and "sugar pills"). Take the first pill of the pack within the first 5 days of your cycle. Take one pill every day until the pack is finished. Then start with the new pack.

**Biphasic/Triphasic pills:**
Different colours indicate hormonal pills of different dosage as well as the placebo pills. Take the first pill of the pack within the first 5 days of your cycle. Take one pill every day until the pack is finished. Then start with the new pack.

**Continous use (exceptional, if advised by health care provider):**
Take pills with hormone contents every day of your cycle and skip the hormone-free interval. This works best with monophasic pills.

# RAGING HORMONES
## Acne and other problems

Women, not just men, produce some male hormones (androgens). Sometimes, they produce too many or they are too active and the following problems may develop:

- Acne
- Oily skin and oily hair (also called seborrhea)
- Excessive hair growth on the face or on other parts of the body (also called hirsutism)

All combined hormonal contraceptives improve acne. Talk to your doctor about OC brands that are specifically approved for treating these problems and still provide reliable contraception just like the other brands:

- Alesse® and Tri-Cyclen®: are helpful in treating mild to moderate acne. If you have severe acne, ask your doctor about Diane-35® which reduces the amount of androgens, reduces the sensitivity of the oil-producing glands to those hormones, and slows down oil production. It works in more than one way and therefore is prescribed for severe cases of acne, oily skin, and excessive hair growth. Diane-35® is not an oral contraceptive but does provide a contraceptive effect. It should not be prescribed for the purpose of birth control alone.

He or she has to know these details about you in order to get a full picture.

The physician may then perform a physical exam with the following:
- check weight and height
- take blood pressure
- breast exam
- pelvic exam (Pap, STI screen)

The pelvic exam can be postponed until the next visit. However, the physician does need to make sure that you are not pregnant and that your blood pressure is okay. At the same time, you may be tested for infections or for pregnancy, if you are at risk. The Pap smear is to look for pre-cancer cells in your cervix, which can be treated. The STI testing is not part of a routine exam and has to be requested. Don't worry – the first pelvic exam is not that big a deal.

### A first prescription gets you started
You may receive a one-month supply of the pill the physician has chosen for you with a prescription for a 6-12 month period. The physician usually asks you to come back after a few months for a check-up or you may call if you have any side effects or bleeding problems. This second visit is a great chance to ask some more questions or to discuss any unwanted effects. Use this opportunity to ask anything that came to mind in the past months. If you have been having problems to take the pill regularly, some OC "starter kits" with tips and reminders to take the pill every day might be helpful.

### Why are there so many different brands?
A great variety of products allow the health care provider to pick the pill that is right for you. Women have different reactions to hormone content and the type of hormones. Sometimes it might take a while until you find the right brand that suits you best. If acne is a problem you might want to talk to your doctor about OCs that treat mild and severe acne. Please refer to the information at the side of the page.

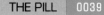 

If bloating is a problem you might want to talk about an OC that minimises water retention.

## Why are there 21-day and 28-day pill packs?

All OCs available at present are based on a 28-day cycle. Most OCs are available in 21-day packs and many are also available as a 28-day pack. In the 28-day pack there are 21 tablets with hormones and 7 tablets without hormones, called placebos. These pills serve as a reminder to take the pill every day. Discard the pack after you have finished the cycle even if you did not take the placebo pills.

## Estrogen content can make a difference

The side effects many women are concerned about are often due to the amount of estrogen in the pill. The amount of estrogen in the most recent OCs varies between 20mcg to 50mcg depending on the brand. All brands that have 35mcg or less of estrogen are called low-dose oral contraceptives. Your physician will likely prescribe you a low-dose preparation. However, estrogen-related side effects usually improve after the first 1-3 cycles of use.

Medical research still continues and development aims for a smaller hormone content, new progestins, and fewer side effects without giving up the high reliability and safety of the method. No single OC brand has been proven to be superior in terms of efficacy, reliability, or side effects.

## Can I choose the brand I want?

Apart from clinical arguments there are also certain preferences you as the patient might have. Discuss with your physician which OC might be best for you.

## Issues surrounding the pill

We will address some concerns, which especially come up in discussions with people who are against things that are artificial, such as "artificial hormones" or even drugs in general. Here is some food for thought:

### The pill is not natural

It contains artificial hormones. However, the hormones used for oral contraceptives are similar to the ones produced by your body. If natural hormones were used for contraception, they would still have to be slightly modified in order to be absorbed by the body. This is basically done during the production process of hormonal contraceptives.

### Smoking

Here comes the truth again...smoking is bad for you whether you take the pill or not. Make it your "increase health and save money" resolution and give it up! The risk of heart attack, stroke and blood clots (cardiovascular disease) is increased in smokers. However, the risk for these diseases involving the arteries and veins is very low in young women. This changes by the age of 35. That is the reason why we recommend stopping the pill at the age of 35 if you continue to smoke. This also applies to nicotine patches or gums used to stop the habit of smoking. They contain nicotine as well and they are as bad. **Basically the pill makes the dangerous habit of smoking more dangerous.** Stopping the pill and continuing to smoke over the age of 35 increases the risk of developing heart disease, stroke and cancer.

### Cardiovascular disease

This is a general term for diseases of the heart and blood vessels (arteries and veins) such as stroke, heart attack, and venous thromboembolism (VTE). There was a big discussion in the early nineties about a certain group of oral contraceptive pills and their effect on the increase of these diseases in users.

Armies of specialists have conducted studies and have held lengthy discussions with the following outcome:

1. Cardiovascular disease is rare among healthy young women.
2. Women over the age of 35 who smoke should not take OCs.
3. Women at **high risk of thrombosis (blood clots in the veins)** should not take OCs. Risk factors are, for example, a family history of thrombosis or a previous thromboembolic event, for example during a pregnancy.
4. Women at **high risk of heart attack, stroke** or **myocardial infarction** should not take OCs. Risk factors are, amongst others, family history, severe high blood pressure and cigarette smoking over age 35.

All of this to say that just the fear of cardiovascular disease alone should not discourage you from using oral contraceptives. If you have no major risk factors you should not worry. But it is important to talk to your doctor about any doubts or fears.

**Cancer**

Boy, this is a big one! Again there are armies of specialists working on finding out the possible effect of hormones on the development of certain cancers. Cancers of the reproductive organs such as cancer of the **breast**, of the lining of the uterus **(endometrium)**, of the **ovaries** and of the **cervix** are very rare among women during their reproductive years. The risk of these cancers rises after menopause.

**Breast cancer:** Women who do not have children or who have had children very late have a higher risk of developing breast cancer. It is still not clear whether the small increase in breast cancer risk associated with the use of the pill is due to the hormones in the pill itself or whether it is due to the fact that the birth of the first child is delayed by the use of the pill. There seems to be no increase in breast cancer risk with longer duration of OC use, with different dosages of estrogen or with different progestins.

You should discuss OC use with your doctor if you have a mother or a sister who developed breast cancer **before** reaching menopause.

**Endometrial cancer:** Good news: the chances of getting this kind of cancer, which affects the lining of the uterus are much lower in users of OCs. The incidence of endometrial cancer is reduced by 50% or more for many years after OC use. Why? The progestin in the pill reduces the thickness of the lining of the uterus (caused by estrogen) and therefore reduces the risk of endometrial cancer.

**Ovarian cancer:** More good news: the chances of developing this kind of cancer are at least 50% lower in women who take the pill. The risk of ovarian cancer decreased with the duration of OC use. The cancer risk is reduced by 10-12% after the first year and by 50% after five years of use. Ovarian cancer risk is linked to the number of cycles of ovulation. Women who do not take OCs and who do not have any children have the highest number of cycles in their lifetime and are at a higher risk of getting this type of cancer. When using an OC the natural cycles are replaced by artificial ones and ovulation does not happen.

**Cervical cancer:** Infection with human papillomavirus (HPV) is the major risk factor for developing cervical cancer. This type of infection is directly related to sexual behaviour, such as the number of sexual partners. The relationship between OC use and the development of cervical cancer is still uncertain.

The Pap smear, which is performed during a regular gynaecological exam, is an excellent tool for the early detection of this form of cancer.

The pill, along with all other contraceptive methods, cannot prevent you from getting breast cancer. The risk rises with age. For example, in 1993 there were seven cases of breast cancer in Canada in the age group 20-24, and there were 1,595 cases in the age group 45-49.

It is a good idea to get into the habit of doing breast self-exams every month and knowing your breasts better. The best time to do the breast self-exam is 7-10 days after the start of your period. Some women do not like it because they are afraid to find something. Yet finding a knot or a lump early is the key to effective treatment.

A WORD ABOUT BREAST SELF-EXAM

## Lifestyle aspects

Here are the features of the pill that might affect your lifestyle:

- **You can determine the time of your periods**
  If you want to go on a holiday and you do not want to menstruate during this time you can simply skip the hormone-free interval. After you have finished your 21 days of hormonal active pills you start right away with the next sequence of 21 hormonal active pills. The so-called continuous use may also be a good idea for women who suffer from pelvic pain, headaches, bloating and breast tenderness during the hormone-free interval. It also improves symptoms associated with endometriosis and polycystic ovary syndrome. Studies have shown no negative health effects for the continuous use of OCs but the long-term effects are still unknown. Irregular bleeding can occur, especially during the first three cycles.

- **You do not have to plan too much ahead**
  Since you take the pill every day you are protected against pregnancy every day. You do not have to plan when to have sex or not to have sex. However, for dual protection, you should have condoms with you in case your partner has not been tested negative for STIs in two tests, six months apart. (Refer to chapter 2)

- **The solution for acne problems**
  Acne comes with growing up and it is one of its most annoying side effects! Acne improves with the use of most combined hormonal contraceptives. Please check out page 38.

- **You have to start a daily routine**
  No benefits without showing some effort! You have to come up with some sort of routine to remember taking the pill DAILY at a certain time. Keep your pack of tablets by your bed, next to your toothbrush or put it in your wallet to make sure you do not forget to take your pill daily. Be creative and think of something! When you plan a holiday away from

home also remember to take your pills with you. It is difficult to get a replacement when you are in Mexico or on a Caribbean island. The names of brands vary from country to country and you might have to see a physician to get a replacement for your prescription away from home. Have an extra pack with you.

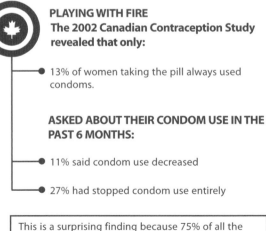

**PLAYING WITH FIRE**
**The 2002 Canadian Contraception Study revealed that only:**

13% of women taking the pill always used condoms.

**ASKED ABOUT THEIR CONDOM USE IN THE PAST 6 MONTHS:**

11% said condom use decreased

27% had stopped condom use entirely

This is a surprising finding because 75% of all the women in the survey who used the pill and condoms together were satisfied with this combined method.

# TROUBLESHOOTING

The following are rare warning signs that should signal you to stop taking the pill and to go directly to the emergency room of a hospital near you:

- **Strong pain in the chest or in the legs;**
- **severe pain in the abdomen;**
- **shortness of breath;**
- **sudden loss of vision or disturbance of vision;**
- **severe headaches; or**
- **yellowing of the skin.**

Here are other signs that are much less serious and do not warrant stopping the pill before talking to your physician. These signs are not hazardous to your health and normally disappear after the first 1-3 cycles of taking the pill. They also do not impair the effectiveness of your OC unless you stop taking it regularly. Never stop taking the pill without talking to your doctor first.

## Irregular bleeding ⚠

Unexpected bleeding (bleeding between hormone-free intervals or spotting) occurs in 10-30% of OC users in the first 3 cycles of use. The body needs to adapt to these new kinds of hormones and it takes a while.

Many studies have been conducted but no single brand of OCs has really proven itself to be the best in preventing irregular bleeding. Use the brand for at least 3-4 cycles. If the problem does not stop, keep on taking the pill and consult your physician again.

## No bleeding at all (amenorrhoea) ⚠

It occurs in 2-3% of cycles. This is nothing to worry about unless you forgot to take the pill or the pill was not absorbed by your body (due to vomiting for example) and you had unprotected intercourse. In this case no bleeding can mean that you are pregnant! Do a pregnancy test but continue the pill daily until you get the result.

## Breast tenderness and nausea ⚠

This is common during the first 3 cycles of OC use and usually improves with time. Taking the pill at bedtime or together with food might help. A pill with a lower estrogen dose may also help.

## Weight gain ⚠

Studies comparing OCs with other methods of contraception failed to show any significant weight gain in OC users. With the use of low-dose pills (35mcg of estrogen content or less), weight gain is minimal and is often due to normal age related weight gain in adolescents. It is possible that during the first months of use an increased appetite may lead to eating more. Keep in mind that healthy diet and regular exercise are the best way to maintain a healthy weight. Water retention can also give the impression of weight gain. You may want to discuss this issue with your physician.

## Mood changes

In most cases irritability or depressed mood have other causes than the use of an OC.

## Chloasma

Chloasma are brown spots on the face, which develop in some women as a response to estrogen. This is due to an overproduction of pigments. The use of a sunscreen prevents the development of chloasma because chloasma can develop as a response to sun exposure – just like tanning! You might have to see a dermatologist if it does not get better.

## Vomiting and diarrhoea

This might make the pill less effective. You should use a backup method of contraception such as the condom during this period and the seven following days.

## Pregnancy

If you become pregnant while taking an OC you should stop taking the pill and consult your physician for a follow-up of the pregnancy. But there is no reason for panic because there is no increased risk of birth defects as a result of OC use during pregnancy.

## Headaches

Headaches, which occur after starting a pill, may be a reason to stop taking it. Consult your physician first. Women who experience headaches during the hormone-free interval can overcome this problem by taking their OC continuously.

## Problem with vision

If you wear contact lenses you may experience some discomfort or change of vision. If this persists you should contact your optometrist for refitting.

## Drug interactions

Always inform your physician about all the drugs you are taking. They might change the action of your birth control pill. Some medications such as certain antibiotics can cause the failure of your OCs in preventing pregnancy. On the other hand, your pill might cause other medications you were prescribed to fail as well. It is important to talk to your health care provider and/or your pharmacist about it. If you have to take a medication, which makes the pill less effective, always use another method of contraception as a backup.

## Missed pills ⚠

No panic...but you will have to use a backup method. Here is how to manage missed pills:

- Missing tablets at the beginning or end of the 21-day cycle has the effect of lengthening the hormone-free interval
- If the hormone-free interval exceeds seven days, the risk of ovulation and possible pregnancy increases
- Forgetting tablets in the second or third week of the 21-day cycle may also increase the risk of ovulation

## INSTRUCTIONS REGARDING MISSED PILLS:

### ➡ For 30-35 mcg ethinylestradiol pills
**Missed 1 or 2 active (hormonal) pills or started a pack 1 or 2 days late**
- Take an active (hormonal) pill a.s.a.p.* and then continue taking pills daily, 1 each day.
- You do not need any additional contraceptive method.

**Missed 3 or more active (hormonal) pills or if started a pack 3 or more days late**
- You should take an active (hormonal) pill a.s.a.p.* and then continue taking pills daily, 1 each day.
- You should also use condoms or abstain from sex until you have taken active (hormonal) pills for 7 days in a row.

**Missed pills in the 3rd week**
- you should finish the active (hormonal) pills in your current pack and start a new pack the next day.
- Do not take the 7 inactive pills.

**Missed pills in the 1st week and had unprotected sex**
- you may want to consider the use of emergency contraception.

### ➡ For 20 mcg or less ethinylestradiol pills
**Missed 1 active (hormonal) pill or started a pack 1 day late**
- Follow the guidance above for "Missed 1 or 2 active (hormonal) pills"

**Missed 2 or more active (hormonal) pills or started a pack 2 or more days late**
- Follow the guidance above for "Missed 3 or more active (hormonal) pills"

### ➡ For all ethinylestradiol pills, regardless of dosage
**Missed any inactive (non-hormonal) pills**
- Discard the missed, inactive (non-hormonal) pills and then continue taking pills daily, 1 pill each day.

\* If you miss more than 1 active (hormonal) pill, take the first missed pill and then either continue taking the rest of the missed pills or discard them to stay on schedule.

Depending on when you remember that you missed a pill(s), take 2 pills on the same day.

**FREQUENTLY ASKED QUESTIONS**

 **Am I too young; am I too old for the pill?**

There is no lower age limit because of the many benefits of the pill, which by far outweigh the risks of an unintended pregnancy. You do not even have to wait until you want to have sex. After you have your first menstrual bleeding the pill can do a great job in helping you to get regular cycles and it can help you to have less pain during your menstruation.

You are also not too old. The recommendation that women should stop taking OCs when they are past 35 is history. Healthy women who do not smoke can take the pill up to menopause.

 **Should I interrupt taking the pill every once in a while?**

Absolutely not. There shouldn't be any interruptions unless you WANT to get pregnant.

 **Will the doctor tell my parents?**

No. Physicians and other health care providers must respect confidentiality.

(?) **When taking a 21-day pill, can I have sex during the hormone-free interval?**

Yes, you are protected all the time, provided you have been taking your pill regularly.

## (?) Will I be able to become pregnant after stopping the pill?

Yes. After stopping the pill you should wait and use other methods of contraception until your first period. This makes it easier to calculate the beginning of a pregnancy.

### Media scare
The OC is the most researched medication that exists. No wonder. It is taken by more than 100 million women across all continents. Because there are so many people still researching and so many women who rely on this type of contraception, media around the world is always very interested in new stories about the pill. If you ever read or hear something scary about the oral contraceptive **do not panic. Continue taking your OC daily and make an appointment to see your doctor who can explain what the problem is all about. Do not stop taking it and risk a pregnancy!**

# TRANSDERMAL CONTRACEPTIVE PATCH

**IN A NUTSHELL**

### Who controls the show?
The woman.

### Does it protect against sexually transmitted infections and HIV?
No.

### What is the patch all about?
EVRA® contains an estrogen and a progestin. It is a patch which needs to be changed every week. It replaces the natural female cycle by an artificial one. The ovaries stop ovulating thus making pregnancy unlikely. The patch also changes the cervical mucus and the lining of the uterus. This "triple action" makes the patch extremely effective in preventing pregnancy.

### What makes this method so special?
- It is a highly effective, reversible method of contraception.
- It is a "less-worry" method because you do not have to take a pill every day.
- Less failures expected because patch users don't have to remember to take a pill every day.
- Probably same non-contraceptive benefits as the combined OC.

### How do I get it?
See a family physician, a gynaecologist, a school nurse or a family planning clinic and ask about EVRA®.

### Possible problems
There might be some unwanted side effects such as irregular bleeding or increased bleeding, breast tenderness, headaches, and nausea. They usually disappear after the first few cycles.

### How effective is the patch in preventing unintended pregnancy?
92-99.7% effective.

### Necessary routine
Change patch weekly.

Actual size

## WHAT IS THE CONTRACEPTIVE PATCH ALL ABOUT?

The patch is the new kid on the block. It has been available since early 2004. The patch contains a progestin (norelgestromin) and an estrogen (ethinylestradiol). Low doses of these hormones are released continuously and absorbed through your skin into your system.

### What non-contraceptive benefits does the contraceptive patch have to offer?

Regular bleeding intervals are the biggest advantage of the patch. It probably offers similar advantages as the combined oral contraceptive pill but no studies have been performed to verify this.

### How does the patch work?

The mechanism of action is the same as the oral contraceptive pill. Instead of taking the necessary estrogen and progestin dose in a tablet, a patch is used. The patch releases 150µg of norelgestromin and 20µg of ethinylestradiol through a membrane in the patch. The hormones are then absorbed by the skin and get into the bloodstream.

### How effective is the patch in preventing unintended pregnancy?

99.7% effective if used correctly. With typical use, eight pregnancies may occur in 100 women who use the method for 12 months. It is as effective as the OC, the contraceptive ring and the POP.

### Does the patch protect against sexually transmitted infections and HIV?

No. The patch does not protect you and your partner from STIs and HIV. The simple recipe for safer sex is to use dual protection! Use a condom (male condom or female condom) for protection against STIs and HIV and get the patch for protection against pregnancy!

### How popular is the patch in Canada?

The patch is a newer contraceptive method. There are no statistics available yet.

### The patch may be a good choice for you if you are looking for a method that...

- requires no day-to-day routine
- is simple and very effective
- is reversible
- is a good alternative to the pill

Basically, the patch may be an option for any woman seeking effective contraception. However,

### The patch is not for you, if...

- you have current or past history of venous thromboembolism (blood clots)
- you have certain cardiovascular conditions
- you suffer from diabetes with end-organ involvement
- you experience headaches with aura
- you were diagnosed with breast cancer
- you have liver disease
- you are pregnant
- you weigh more than 90kg

## Where do I get the patch?

You should make an appointment with your family physician, a gynaecologist, a school nurse, a public health clinic, or a family planning clinic. The interview and the health check-up are the same as with the pill. Please refer to page 34. Some health services provide the patch without a prescription. You will be asked to go for a check-up to obtain the prescription later.

## Which contraceptive patches are available in Canada?

EVRA® is the only brand available in Canada. Although contraceptive patches are recent, hormonal patches have been used for many years to treat menopausal symptoms.

## How do I get started?

1. A first-day start is recommended.
2. Apply a patch on the first day of your menses to clean, dry, healthy and intact skin. Choose one of the following sites: buttock, abdomen, upper outer arm, upper torso. Do not apply the patch on the breast. This is the "patch change day".
3. After one week, remove the patch and apply a new one. It should be the same day of the week as the day when you first applied a patch.
4. In total you use 3 patches in 3 weeks. The fourth week is hormone-free or "patch-free". During this time you will experience bleeding (your period).
5. Check daily whether the patch is still in place.

The patch is effective from the day you first use it when you choose the first day start. If you start later in your cycle (for example on the second day of bleeding) you have to use a back-up method for seven days if you have sex.

## ISSUES SURROUNDING THE CONTRACEPTIVE PATCH

### What do I do if the patch falls off?

If the patch has fallen off either partly or completely for less than 24 hours, try to reattach the patch. If it does not stick, remove it and put a new patch on. Keep the usual patch change day. If the patch has been off for more than 24 hours, apply a new patch and use a back-up method for 1 week if you have sex.

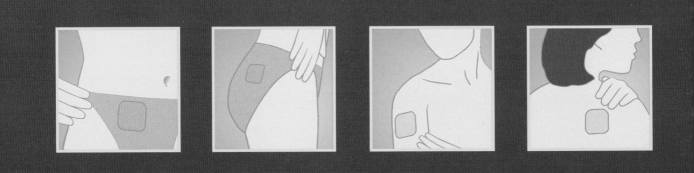

## What do I do if I forget to change or apply a patch?

It depends when this happens during your cycle.

**Week 1:** If you forget to apply the patch in week 1, you are increasing the hormone-free interval and you are at risk of getting pregnant. Apply the patch immediately and use back-up method for 1 week if you have sex.

**Week 2 or 3:** If you are **less than 48 hours** late applying your new patch, apply it as soon as you remember. No back-up method needed.

If you are **more than 48 hours** late, apply your new patch and start a new cycle. You will need back-up contraception for one week if you have sex.

**Week 4:** This is supposed to be the patch-free week. If you forgot to remove the patch, remove it as soon as you remember. Apply the next new patch on the usual "patch-change day".

The hormone-free interval, or "patch-free interval", should never be more than 7 days long.

## Does the patch stick during exercise and showering?

The patch sticks really well. It is unlikely that it will come off even in the toughest conditions such as saunas, whirlpools, or while swimming.

## What about weight gain?

Studies could not find any weight changes related to the use of the contraceptive patch.

## Continuous Use

As with the birth control pill, continuous use of the patch may help women who suffer from pelvic pain, headaches, bloating and breast tenderness during the hormone free interval (patch free week). You may want to discuss this option with your health care provider.

# TROUBLESHOOTING

Sometimes women worry because they have side effects that they weren't expecting. Some of these side effects are common and often disappear after the first three months of use.

### Irregular bleeding

Irregular bleeding is a common complaint during the first few months of use of any hormonal contraceptive method. Studies have shown that irregular bleeding in patch users is similar to that seen with the pill. The bleeding usually improves with time. If the bleeding continues after the first few months, discuss with your health care provider.

### Breast symptoms and headaches

Breast symptoms during the first 3 cycles of patch use are more common than they are with the pill. Again, these symptoms usually improve with time. Only few patients discontinue the patch because of headaches.

### Local skin reaction

Up to 20% of users may experience local skin reactions, which are usually mild or moderate in nature. Less than 2% of patch users have to stop using the patch because of a skin reaction. Changing application sites every week may help.

### Drug interactions

Always inform your physician about all the drugs you are taking.

# CONTRACEPTIVE RING

### Who controls the show?
The woman.

### What is the vaginal ring all about?
NuvaRing® contains an estrogen and a progestin and is inserted in the vagina where it stays for three weeks. It replaces the natural female cycle by an artificial one. The ovaries stop producing eggs and there is no ovulation. The ring's action also changes the mucus in the cervix and the lining of the uterus. This "triple action" makes the ring extremely effective in preventing pregnancy.

### How do I get it?
See a family physician, a gynaecologist, a school nurse or a family planning clinic and ask about NuvaRing®.

### How effective is the ring in preventing unintended pregnancy?
92-99.7% effective.

### Does it protect against sexually transmitted infections and HIV?
No.

### What makes this method so special?
- It is a highly effective, reversible method of contraception.
- It is a "less-worry" method because you do not have to follow a daily pill-taking routine.
- Less failures expected because ring users don't have to remember to take a pill every day.
- Probably same non-contraceptive benefits as the combined OC.

### Possible problems
There might be some side effects such as irregular bleeding or increased bleeding, breast tenderness, headaches, and nausea. They usually disappear after the first few cycles.

### Necessary routine
Remove ring every three weeks.

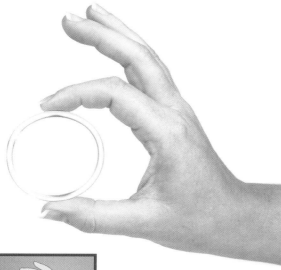

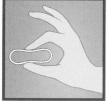

### WHAT IS THE CONTRACEPTIVE RING ALL ABOUT?

The ring is another new contraceptive available in Canada since early 2005. The ring contains a progestin (etonogestrel) and an estrogen (ethinylestradiol). These hormones are released from the ring on a daily basis, and low doses are absorbed by your system through the vaginal mucosa.

### What non-contraceptive benefits does the contraceptive ring have to offer?

It probably offers similar advantages as the combined oral contraceptive pill but no studies have been performed to prove benefits other than reliable contraception.

### How does the ring work?

The mechanism of action is the same as the oral contraceptive pill. Instead of taking the necessary estrogen and progestin dose in a tablet, a vaginal ring is used. Every day, it releases 120µg of etonogestrel and 15µg of ethinylestradiol through the membrane of the ring when placed in the vagina. The hormones are then absorbed through the vaginal mucosa and get into the bloodstream.

### How effective is the ring in preventing unintended pregnancy?

99.7% effective if used correctly. The ring is as effective as the OC, the POP and the contraceptive patch. The "user failure rate" is about 8%. Perfect compliance is seen in 85.6 to 91% of contraceptive ring users, which is much higher than with pill users.

### Does the ring protect against sexually transmitted infections and HIV?

No. The ring does not protect you and your partner from STIs and HIV. The simple recipe for safer sex is to use dual protection! Use a condom (male condom or female condom) for protection against STIs and HIV and get the ring for protection against pregnancy! Spermicides do not appear to affect the effectiveness of the ring.

### How popular is the ring in Canada?

The ring is a new contraceptive method and has only been available since January 2005. There are no statistics available yet.

### The contraceptive ring may be a good choice for you if you are looking for a method that...

- requires no day-to-day routine
- is simple and very effective
- is reversible
- is a good alternative for women looking for an alternative to the pill

Basically, the ring may be an option for any woman seeking effective contraception. However,

### The ring is not for you, if...

- you have current or past history of venous thromboembolism (blood clots)
- you have certain cardiovascular conditions
- you suffer from diabetes with end-organ involvement
- you experience migraine headaches with aura
- you were diagnosed with breast cancer, cancer of the endometrium or cervix
- you suffer from vaginal bleeding other than your normal periods
- you have liver disease
- you are pregnant
- you are allergic to any of the components of the ring

### Where do I get NuvaRing®?

You need to make an appointment with your family physician, a gynaecologist or a family planning clinic. You can also contact the health service in your school. The interview and the health check-up are the same as with the pill. Please refer to page 34.

### Which contraceptive rings are available in Canada?

NuvaRing® is the only brand available in Canada.

## ISSUES SURROUNDING THE CONTRACEPTIVE RING

### Will I feel the ring and or will my partner feel the ring during intercourse?

If the ring is placed correctly, it is unlikely that you will feel the ring. Some women or their partners will notice the ring during intercourse but this does not usually cause any problems or concerns.

### What do I do if the ring falls out?

It depends on how much time has passed since the ring has fallen out.

If the ring fell out less than three hours ago, rinse it with cool to lukewarm water (not hot water!) and reinsert it.

If more than three hours have passed, rinse the ring, reinsert it, and use a back-up method for seven days if you have sex.

### What happens if I forget to take it out after three weeks?

The ring is actually effective for up to four weeks so this is not a problem. Just take the ring out as soon as you remember. Wait 7 days and then insert a new one. If the ring was in the vagina for more than 4 weeks, pregnancy should be ruled out and you should use a back-up method for seven days if you have sex.

The hormone-free interval, also known as the "ring-free interval", should never be more than 7 days.

# TROUBLESHOOTING

**Sometimes women worry because they have side effects that they weren't expecting. Some of these side effects are common and often disappear after the first three months of use.**

### Unscheduled bleeding or no bleeding

Breakthrough bleeding and spotting are common complaints during the first few months of use of any hormonal contraceptive method. Ring users may in fact have less irregular bleeding than combined OC users, especially in the first cycle of use.

### Breast symptoms and headaches

In clinical studies about 5.8% of ring users experienced headaches, 3.2% nausea, and 2.6% breast tenderness. These problems usually diminish after a few months of use.

### Vaginal symptoms

The most common local side effects of using the ring are vaginitis (an inflammation of the vagina) and leukorrhea (an increase in vaginal secretions). These occurred in less than 6% of ring users. For most women, PAP test results remained normal after 1 year of ring use.

### Drug interactions ⚠

Always inform your physician about all the drugs you are taking.

## How do I get started?

1. Read the "how to start" section of the package insert booklet.
2. Make use of the stickers at the back of this booklet and the timer the manufacturer is offering.
3. Call your doctor immediately if certain problems occur. Like any other medication, side effects can occur, which need immediate attention. In your package insert booklet you can read about these warning signs.

## How do I get the routine, how to remember?

The ring is inserted and left in place for 3 weeks and then removed for 1 week (the ring-free interval). Withdrawal bleeding usually occurs during the ring-free interval. The ring-free interval should be no longer than 7 days.

If you were not using a hormonal contraceptive in the previous month, the first ring cycle is started between day 1 and day 5 of the menstrual cycle. During the first cycle, an additional barrier method of contraception, such as condoms is recommended until after the first seven days of continuous ring use.

## Switch from another method

To switch from the combined OC to the vaginal ring, the ring should be inserted no later than 7 days after the last combined OC tablet was taken (the tablets that contain the hormones). No back-up method is needed.

To switch from a progestin-only pill, the vaginal ring is inserted the day after the last pill is taken. An additional barrier method of contraception, such as condoms should be used for the first seven days after the ring is inserted.

To switching from an injectable contraceptive method, the ring is inserted on the day when the next injection would be due. An additional barrier method of contraception, such as condoms, should be used for the first seven days after the ring is inserted.

## Travel

Women who are travelling across different time zones for business or pleasure don't need to worry about adjusting their pill-taking timing - the ring is already in place and travels with them.

## Continuous use

If you want to go on a holiday and you do not want to menstruate during this time you can simply skip the ring-free interval. After you have finished your 3 weeks of ring use you start right away with a new ring for an additional 3 weeks. As with the pill, "continuous use" may also help women who suffer from pelvic pain, headaches, and bloating and breast tenderness during the hormone-free interval. It also improves symptoms associated with endometriosis and polycystic ovary syndrome. One clinical study found no negative health effects when the ring was used continuously, but the long-term effects are still unknown. Irregular bleeding can occur, especially during the first three cycles.

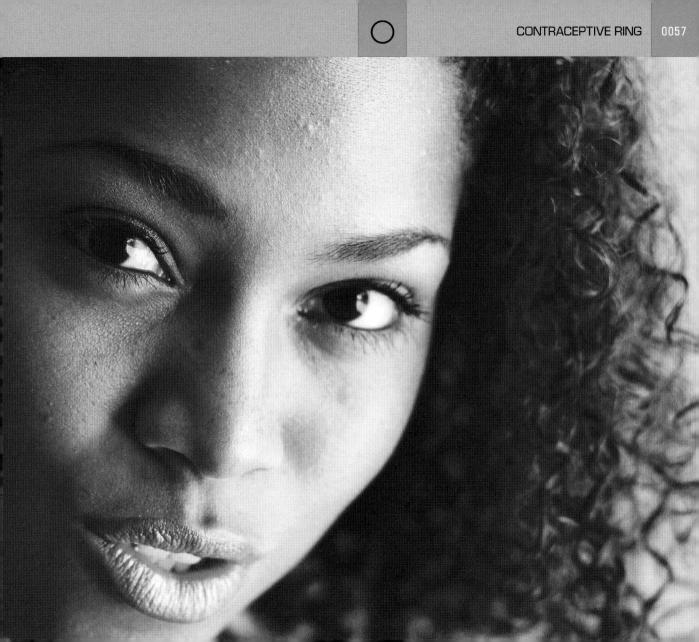

# PROGESTIN-ONLY PILL (POP)

**IN A NUTSHELL**

**Who controls the show?**
The woman.

**Does it protect against sexually transmitted infections and HIV?**
No.

**What is the POP all about?**
The POP, also known as the "mini pill" contains one hormone, a progestin. It interferes with the natural cycle but the ovaries keep working. The progestin acts on the lining of the uterus walls and on the mucus at the entrance of the cervix to make it difficult for sperm to get through. The POP also inhibits ovulation in 60% of users. You have to take the POP **every day at the same** time. There is NO hormone-free interval.

**What makes this method so special?**
- It is a highly effective, reversible method of contraception.
- It may be used by women who are otherwise not allowed to use the pill because of certain health problems or because they can't take estrogen.
- It can be used by breastfeeding women.
- It offers additional health benefits such as reduced menstrual pain and menstrual blood flow and protection against certain cancers.

**How do I get it?**
See a family physician, a gynaecologist, a school nurse or a family planning clinic and ask about Micronor®.

**Possible problems**
- Forgetting pills. This method is not very forgiving if you don't take the pills at the same time every day.
- Irregular bleeding.

**How effective is the POP in preventing unintended pregnancy?**
92-99.7% effective.

**Necessary routine**
Take pill daily at the same time.

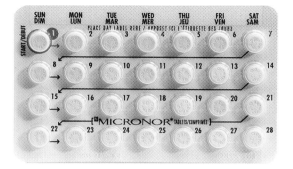

## WHAT IS THE POP ALL ABOUT?

The Progestin-only Pill (POP) is a birth control pill which contains only one hormone: a progestin. This method is only for women who can remember to take a pill <u>every day at the same time</u>. This pill allows for no error in pill taking because it contains only one hormone and can only prevent unintended pregnancy when taken absolutely regularly. It is also a good choice for women who are breast-feeding. There is only one brand available in Canada, which is called Micronor®. It contains 35mcg of Norethindrone.

### What non-contraceptive benefits does the POP have to offer?
The POP:
- reduces menstrual flow
- induces amenorrhea (no periods) in 10% of users
- reduces menstrual and pre-menstrual pain

### How does the POP work?
The hormone progestin in the POP sends messages to the brain and to the sex organs to change the lining of the uterus. This lining, known as the endometrium, becomes unfriendly for an egg to settle in and develop. It also changes the mucus at the entrance to the cervix. This mucus becomes thicker and more difficult for the sperm to go through.

Unlike the oral contraceptive pill, the POP does not fully prevent ovulation. Ovulation will still occur in 40% of all cycles.

### How effective is the POP in preventing unintended pregnancy?
This method is 99.7% effective if used correctly. It is as effective as the OC, the ring and the patch if taken correctly, meaning absolutely regularly, at the same time of day, every day! The failure rate for typical use is around 8%.

### Does the POP protect against sexually transmitted infections and HIV?

No. The POP does not protect you and your partner from STIs and HIV. The simple recipe for safer sex is to use dual protection! Use a condom (male latex condom or female condom) for protection against STIs and HIV and use the POP for protection against pregnancy!

### The POP is a good choice for you, if you are looking for a method that...

- is very reliable
- has no estrogen-related side effects
- makes your periods lighter
- you can stop any time if you want to have a baby
- offers certain additional health benefits
- is a good alternative for women
  - who are over the age of 35 and still smoke
  - who suffer from migraine headaches
  - who are breast-feeding
  - who suffer from sickle cell disease

Basically, the POP may be an option for any woman seeking effective contraception. However,

### The POP is not for you, if...

- you cannot remember to take a pill at the same time every day
- you cannot tolerate irregular bleeding
- you are already pregnant
- you suffer from vaginal bleeding other than your period
- you have breast cancer

### Where do I get the POP?

You need to make an appointment with your family physician, a gynaecologist, a school nurse or at a family planning clinic. The interview and the health check-up are the same as with the pill. Please refer to page 34.

## ISSUES SURROUNDING THE POP

### Breastfeeding / after delivery of a baby

The POP can be taken right after the delivery of the baby. If the woman chooses to breastfeed, the POP will not have any effect on the quality or quantity of the breast milk.

### Cardiovascular disease, heart attacks, and stroke

The POP does not increase the risk of cardiovascular disease, heart attack, or stroke. In fact, the POP is a choice for women with a past history of venous thromboembolism (blood clots) and women who have a higher risk of myocardial infarction and stroke.

# HOW DO I GET STARTED?

You will receive a one month supply of the POP and a prescription for usually a year. The physician might ask you to come back after three months for a check-up. This second visit is a great chance to ask some more questions or to discuss any unwanted effects. Use this opportunity to ask anything that came to mind in the past three months.

### How do I take my POP, how do I remember?

**1** Study the package insert. It sounds like a boring idea but...the package inserts of contraceptives are the best package inserts available. They tell you a lot about the POP.

**2** Make use of the stickers with the days on it to remember to take a tablet daily.

**3** Call your doctor immediately if certain problems occur. As with any other medication, side effects can occur which need immediate attention. In your package insert you can read about these warning signs.

### Use the Day 1 start.

As a new starter you should choose the "Day 1 start". On the first day of your cycle, which is the first day of bleeding, you take the first pill in the pack. After that you continue to take one pill every day until the pack is finished. Then you immediately start the next pack. **With the POP there is no hormone-free interval like with the combined oral contraceptive**. Make it a daily routine to take one pill at the same time every day. Do not go more than three hours past your regular pill taking time or the pill will not be as effective.

**IMPORTANT: During the first seven days you have to use a backup method of contraception such as the male or the female condom because the POP takes a while to become fully effective in preventing pregnancy.**

# TROUBLESHOOTING

Sometimes women stop taking the POP because they have side effects that they weren't expecting. Some of these side effects are common and often disappear after the first three months. We advise you not to stop taking the POP before you have talked to your physician about the problems.

## Missed pills

If a pill is forgotten or vomited, take a pill as soon as possible. Take the next pill at the scheduled time even if you have to take two pills at once. A backup method must be used for at least 48 hours.

If you missed two pills in a row, you must take two pills for two days. A backup method must be used for at least 48 hours.

## Unscheduled bleeding

The likelihood of unscheduled bleeding is higher in the first three months of the use of the POP. In fact, spotting occurs in 12% of users in the first month and decreases over time.

## No bleeding at all (amenorrhoea)

This is very possible with the use of the POP. This is nothing to worry about unless you forgot to take the pill or the pill did not get absorbed by the body (due to vomiting, flu-like illness, diarrhoea, drug interaction) and had unprotected intercourse. In this case no bleeding can mean that you are pregnant! Do a pregnancy test but continue taking the pill daily until you get your results.

## Nausea

This is uncommon with this kind of pill. Taking the POP at bedtime or with food might help.

## Vomiting

Vomiting might make the pill less effective. You should use a backup method of contraception such as the condom for seven days.

## Pregnancy

If you become pregnant while taking the POP you should stop taking it immediately. But there is no reason for panic because there is no increased risk of birth defects as a result of POP use during pregnancy.

## Drug interactions

Always inform your physician about all the drugs you are taking. They might change the action of your POP. Some medications can cause the failure of your pill in preventing pregnancy. On the other hand your POP might cause other medications you were prescribed to fail as well. It is important to talk to your health care provider and/or your pharmacist about it.

# INJECTABLE CONTRACEPTIVE

**Who controls the show?**
The woman.

**Does it protect against sexually transmitted infections and HIV?**
No.

**What is the injectable contraceptive all about?**
It contains one hormone, a progestin. It interferes with the natural cycle, but does not completely replace it like the pill does. It stops ovulation and acts on the lining of the uterus walls and on the mucus at the entrance of the cervix to make it difficult for sperm to get through.

**What makes this method so special?**
- It is one of the most effective reversible methods of contraception.
- It is a "less-worry" method because you do not have to follow a daily pill-taking routine.
- It can be used by women who cannot take estrogen due to certain health conditions.
- It provides contraception for 12 weeks.
- It offers additional health benefits.

**How do I get it?**
See a family physician, a gynaecologist, a school nurse or a family planning clinic and ask about Depo-Provera®.

**Possible problems**
Bleeding irregularities, decrease in bone mineral density (BMD) and weight gain are possible concerns with this method. 50% of women stop their periods altogether within one year of use.

**How effective is the injection in preventing unintended pregnancy?**
97-99.7% effective.

**Necessary routine**
Go for the injection every 12 weeks.

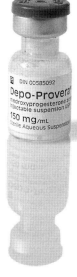

- Decreases the incidence of seizures and cyclic headaches
- Possibly reduces the risk of pelvic inflammatory disease and incidence of sickle cell crisis.

### How does the injectable contraceptive work?

The hormone progestin (medroxyprogesterone acetate) sends messages to the brain and to the sex organs to stop the monthly release of an egg (ovulation). The endometrium also becomes unfriendly for an egg to settle in and develop if ovulation occurs. It also changes the mucus at the entrance to the cervix. This mucus becomes thicker and makes it more difficult for the sperm to move and travel to the uterus.

### How effective is the injection in preventing unintended pregnancy?

This method is 99.7% effective if used perfectly. In other words: In 1000 women who used the method for 1 year, only 3 pregnancies were reported. This method is one of the most effective reversible methods of contraception, comparable in effectiveness with the pill, the POP, the ring and the patch. The failure rate for typical use is 3%.

### Does the injection protect against sexually transmitted infections and HIV?

No. The injection does not protect you and your partner from STIs. The simple recipe for safer sex is to use dual protection! Use a condom (male latex condom or female condom) for protection against STIs and HIV and get the injection for protection against pregnancy!

### How popular is the injection in Canada?

In the 2002 Canadian Contraception Study, the injection was used by 2% of all women who responded to the questionnaire.

## WHAT IS THE INJECTABLE CONTRACEPTIVE ALL ABOUT?

The injectable contraceptive is given once every 10-13 weeks (four times a year). It contains only one hormone, a progestin. It is available in Canada since 1997 under the name Depo-Provera®.

### What non-contraceptive benefits does the injectable contraceptive have to offer?

Injectable contraceptive:

- Induces amenorrhea (no bleeding) in over 55% of women after one year of using the method
- Reduces the risk of endometrial cancer
- Reduces symptoms of endometriosis, premenstrual syndrome, and chronic pelvic pain

**The injectable contraceptive may be a good choice for you, if you are looking for a method that...**

- is simple and very effective
- requires no day-to-day routine
- does not contain estrogen
- is long-lasting (10-13 weeks)
- makes your periods lighter; in 50% of women the periods will stop within one year of use
- offers certain additional health benefits

It is a good alternative for women who

- cannot take the pill due to the estrogen
- who have a problem with taking the pill or the Progestin-only pill on a daily basis
- who are over the age of 35 and still smoke
- who suffer from migraine headaches
- who are breast-feeding
- who suffer from sickle cell disease
- who suffer from endometriosis
- who take anti-seizure medication

Basically, the injection may be an option for any woman seeking effective contraception. However,

**The injection is not for you, if...**

- you are already pregnant
- you suffer from unexplained vaginal bleeding other than your period
- you suffer from a severe liver disease
- you cannot tolerate bleeding irregularities
- you cannot make regular appointments every 12 to 13 weeks for a follow-up injection
- you want to get pregnant quickly after stopping your birth control method

### Where do I get the injection?

You need to make an appointment with your family physician, a gynaecologist, a school nurse or at a family planning clinic. The interview and the health check-up are the same as with the pill. Please refer to page 34.

### What to expect during the procedure.

You get an injection into a muscle in the upper arm, buttocks or thigh. Make an appointment for your next visit in 10-13 weeks immediately. That way you will not forget!

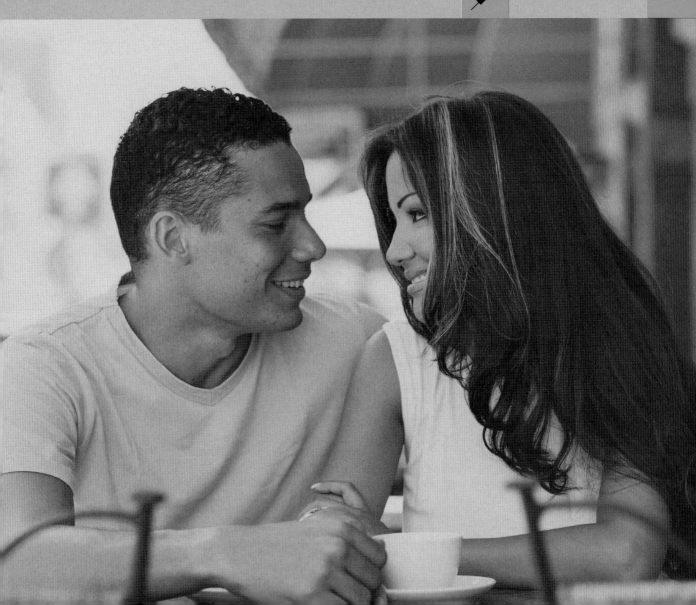

Try to time your visit so that you can get the injection during the first five days of your menstrual cycle, meaning during the first few days of bleeding. Depo-Provera® is fully effective in preventing pregnancy 24 hours after it is given. No backup method is required.

If you do not or cannot (example: you have no periods for a while) receive Depo-Provera® during the first 5 days of a normal menstrual period, you should have a pregnancy test to ensure that you are not pregnant. You should use another contraceptive method as a backup for a minimum of 1 week following the injection.

## ISSUES SURROUNDING THE INJECTABLE CONTRACEPTIVE

### Breastfeeding / after delivery of a baby
A woman can have her first injection immediately after delivering the baby. It is safe to breastfeed while using Depo-Provera® because the progestin has no effect on the quality and quantity of breast milk.

### Decreased bone density
Studies have shown that women who use Depo-Provera® will experience a decrease in bone mineral density (BMD). BMD is an indicator for healthy bones. In adolescents, the decrease in BMD may have a negative effect on achieving peak bone mass. Once the medication is stopped, the bones return partly or even fully to their previous bone density. Exercise, adequate calcium intake, and avoiding smoking will also help to keep your bones healthy. You should discuss this with your physician to find out whether this could be a problem for you.

### Cardiovascular disease, heart attack, and stroke
The injection contraceptive does not increase the risk of cardiovascular disease, heart attack, or stroke. In fact, the injection may be a choice for women with a past history of venous tromboembolism (blood clots) and those who have a higher risk of heart attack or stroke.

### Return to fertility
With the injection, the return to fertility takes longer than with the pill. Once you have had the injection, it is effective for 12 weeks. After the 12 weeks, it may take an average of six months to ovulate and return to your natural cycle again. Studies found that ten months after the last injection, 50% of women who wanted to become pregnant were pregnant. Two years after the last injection, 90% of women that wanted to get pregnant had gotten pregnant.

## TROUBLESHOOTING

**Here are some side effects, which may cause concern and discomfort in women. These effects normally stop after the first few months of use.**

### Unscheduled bleeding or no bleeding

This is one of the big concerns in women using the injection. Many women will experience unpredictable bleeding or spotting following the first two injections (6 months). This problem usually improves over time. Some women stop bleeding altogether within the first year of use. In fact, at 12 months 55-60% of women have no periods and at 24 months 68% of women will have no periods. If bleeding irregularities bother you, do not hesitate to talk to your doctor. There are several ways to deal with this problem.

### Weight gain

This is thought to be due to increased appetite caused by the progestin in the injection. It happens to about 50% of women. Women who gain weight gain approximately 2.5 kg in the first year of use, 3.7 kg after the second year, and 6.3 kg after the fourth year. If you gain weight, rule out other causes such as change in diet, lack of physical activity or other medications, and maintain good eating habits and regular exercise.

### Hormonal side effects and mood changes

Headaches are one of the most common side effects with this method, occurring in 17% of users. Mood changes may occur but may have different origins.

### Drug interactions

Always inform your physician about all the drugs you are taking. Only two medications are known to decrease the effectiveness of the injection.

### Late for the next appointment

You should schedule your appointments in 12-week intervals. The injection of progestin is a reliable contraceptive for up to 13 weeks.

If you cannot make it to the next appointment on time you have to use a backup method of contraception such as the condom (male or female condom) for two weeks. At your next visit you will have to do a pregnancy test before getting the next injection. You will find more details in the patient information that you will receive when getting your first injection.

# IMPLANT

**IN A NUTSHELL**

**Who controls the show?**
The woman.

**What are implants all about?**
Implants contain one hormone, a progestin. It stops ovulation and acts on the lining of the uterus walls and on the mucus at the entrance of the cervix to make it difficult for sperm to get through.

**How do I get it?**
Norplant® is no longer available in Canada. A new product, Implanon®, will be available in the future. See a family physician, a gynaecologist, a school nurse or a family planning clinic.

**How effective are implants in preventing unintended pregnancy?**
99.95% effective.

**Does it protect against sexually transmitted infections and HIV?**
No.

**What makes this method so special?**
- It **is the most effective** reversible method of contraception.
- It is a "no-worry" method because you do not have to follow a daily pill-taking routine.
- It can be used by women who cannot take estrogen.
- Norplant® provides contraception for up to 5 years, Implanon® for up to 3 years.

**Possible problems**
Bleeding irregularities, weight changes. These problems are less frequent with the implant than they are with the injection.

## WHAT ARE IMPLANTS ALL ABOUT?

The implant called Norplant® consisted of six match-sized plastic rods, which were inserted beneath the skin under the upper arm. The rods are 34 mm long, and 2.4 mm in diameter. The rods released a constant dose of the progestin levonorgestrel and provided effective contraception for up to 5 years. Norplant was removed from the market in 2002 and is no longer available. Some women who had it inserted several years ago may still be using it.

The implant called Implanon® has only one rod (40 mm long and 2mm in diameter) instead of six rods with the progestin etonogestrel. This product will be launched in the near future. Implanon® provides contraception for up to three years.

Implants offer additional health benefits, known as "non-contraceptive benefits". Please refer to page 35.

### How do implants work?

The progestin in the implants sends messages to the brain and to the sex organs to change the lining of the uterus. The lining, known as the endometrium, becomes unfriendly for an egg to settle in and develop. It also changes the mucus at the entrance of the cervix. This mucus becomes thicker, which makes it more difficult for the sperm to get through. Implants may also prevent ovulation, especially in the first two years of use.

### How effective are implants in preventing unintended pregnancy?

This method is the most effective reversible method of contraception. It is 99.95% effective. Implanon® is even more effective. In 70,000 cycles of use, not a single pregnancy was reported.

## Do implants protect against sexually transmitted infections and HIV?

No, implants do not protect you and your partner from STIs and HIV. The simple recipe for safer sex is to use dual protection! Use a condom (male latex condom or female condom) for protection against STIs and HIV and get the implant for protection against pregnancy!

**Implants may be a good choice for you if you are looking for a method that...**
- is simple and very effective
- requires no day-to-day routine
- contains no estrogen
- lasts for a number of years
- makes your periods lighter or even disappear
- is a good alternative for women who have a problem with taking the combined oral contraceptive pill or the progestin-only pill on a daily basis

Basically, the implant may be a good option for women looking for an effective, longer term birth control method. However,

**Implants are not for you, if...**
- you cannot tolerate bleeding irregularities
- you are afraid of any weight gain due to increased appetite
- you are afraid of even small surgical procedures (this is necessary for implant and removal)
- you are already pregnant

**Q. I still have Norplant® inserted but I heard it was withdrawn from the market. Should I get the rods removed?**

A. No. The fact that Norplant® is no longer available does not mean that it is less safe or effective. The implant is effective for 5 years. In women weighing less than 70 kg the implant is effective for 7 years.

**Q. I am using Norplant® and I do not have periods. Is that normal?**

A. Yes. About 12% of Norplant® users will experience amenorrhea. With the new implant, Implanon®, this no-bleeding rate will be higher.

**Q. If I decide to become pregnant, how long will it take until my fertility returns?**

A. Ask your physician to remove the implants at any time. On average it takes a woman 1-3 months to resume her normal cycle following the removal of the implant.

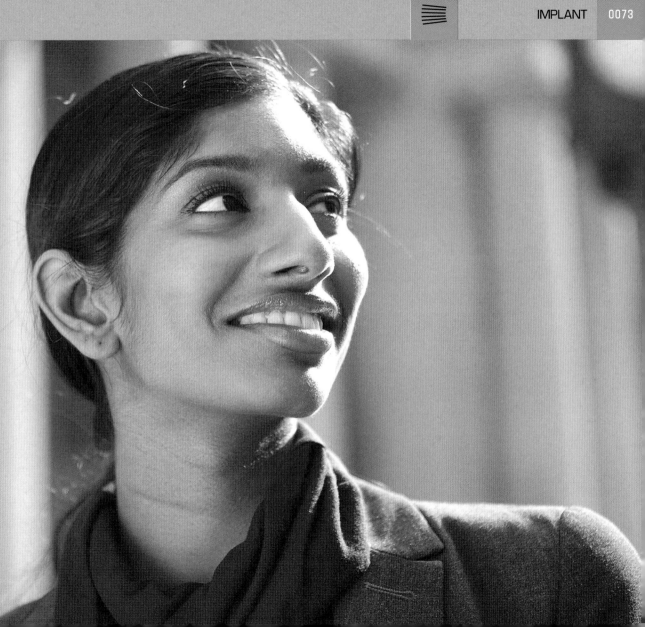

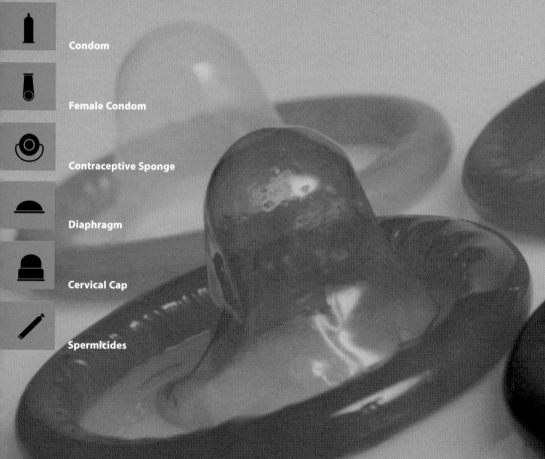

This chapter is about the following methods:

**Condom**

**Female Condom**

**Contraceptive Sponge**

**Diaphragm**

**Cervical Cap**

**Spermicides**

# BARRIER METHODS
## KEYS TO SAFER SEX

The biggest advantage of barrier methods is their role in the **prevention of sexually transmitted infections**. The female condom and male latex condoms are the best performers when it comes to STI and HIV protection. They are the only available contraceptives that offer very good protection against these infections. As you will find out by reading this chapter, other barrier methods offer some protection against STIs as well.

Here are some additional features of barrier methods:

- **Barrier methods do not prevent pregnancy as effectively as hormonal, surgical methods and the IUD or IUS, but they can be used in combination to practice safer sex for dual protection.** Combinations could be:
  - pill and condom
  - IUD or IUS and condom
  - male condom and sponge or spermicide
  - male condom and diaphragm
- **Barrier methods are very convenient:** no doctor's appointment needed (except for the fitting of a diaphragm or cap) and you only use the method when you actually have sex.
- **Barrier methods target sperm:** one way to target sperm is to create a barrier so that male sperm cannot reach the uterus and then the fallopian tubes where there might be an egg waiting to be fertilized. The other way is to destroy sperm upon contact, which is done by spermicides or the sponge, which contains spermicides.
- **Barrier methods have no systemic effects on your body:** they do not interfere with how your body functions.
- **Barrier methods require practice** to use them correctly and need to be used each time you have intercourse.

In the 2002 Canadian Contraception Study, 22% of the respondents were using barrier methods of contraception. The following table gives you a summary of the most popular barrier methods.

**COMPARE AND DECIDE:**
**Barrier Methods of Contraception**

| | Condom | Female Condom |
|---|---|---|
| **Nature of the method** | Barrier | Barrier |
| **Physician appointment necessary** | No | No |
| **Spermicide needed at time of insertion** | No | No |
| **Additional spermicide needed for each new act of intercourse** | No | No |
| **Can be used during menstruation** | Yes | Yes |
| **When to insert/apply** | Rolled over erect penis before intercourse | Anytime before intercourse |
| **When to remove** | After ejaculation | After intercourse and before standing up |
| **Safety: MAXIMUM TIME device can be left in place** | As long as the penis is erect. Once ejaculation has occurred, the penis should be withdrawn while it is still erect. | 8 hours |
| **The device is good for** | Only 1 application | Only 1 application |
| **If lubricant is desired** | Only water-based with latex condom, any lubricant with polyurethane condom | Water- or oil-based |

| Contraceptive sponge | Diaphragm* | Cervical cap* | Spermicides* |
|---|---|---|---|
| Barrier and spermicide in one product | Barrier | Barrier | Chemical to destroy sperm |
| No | Yes | Yes | No |
| No | Yes | Yes | N/A |
| No | Yes, with applicator | Yes, with applicator | Yes |
| No | Yes | No | Yes |
| Can be inserted hours before, but at least 15 minutes before | Anytime before intercourse | Anytime before intercourse | Depending on the product, see chapter 4 |
| No less than 6 hours after intercourse | No less than 6 hours after intercourse | No less than 6 hours after intercourse | N/A |
| 12 hours after it has been inserted | 24 hours after it has been inserted | 3 days | N/A |
| Only 1 application | Reuse for one year or longer | Reuse for one year or longer | 1-24 hours, depending on the product |
| Only water-based | Only water-based with latex diaphragm, any lubricant with silicone | Water- or oil-based with silicone cap | Not necessary |

* Should only be used in monogamous relationships

# CONDOM

**Who controls the show?**
The man.

**What is the condom all about?**
A latex, polyurethane or sheep membrane sheath, which is rolled over the penis. The condom acts as a barrier. It prevents the exchange of body fluids and semen. The latex and polyurethane condoms protect against most STIs and HIV, and against pregnancy. The sheep membrane condom protects only against pregnancy. If the condom is the only contraceptive method used it can be combined with a separate spermicide in a monogamous relationship. Otherwise dual protection is recommended: the female partner should use another method of contraception.

**How do I get it?**
Prescription-free, in vending machines, drugstores, condom shops, on-line...

**How do I use it?**
You roll it on the erect penis before intercourse.

**If you use a lubricant**
Only water-based lubricants for latex condoms.
Any lubricant for the polyurethane condoms.

**How effective is the condom in preventing unintended pregnancy?**
85-98% effective.

**Does the condom protect against sexually transmitted infections and HIV?**
Yes, but not 100%. Latex and polyurethane condoms protect against STIs and HIV with the exception of Herpes and HPV.

Sheep membrane condoms do not protect against STIs and HIV.

**What makes the condom so special?**
- It can be used in combination with other methods to practice safer sex and to get dual protection.
- The condom has benefits other than protection against pregnancy: latex and polyurethane condoms protect against most STIs and HIV.
- All condoms can become part of foreplay and can improve sexual relations.

**Possible problems**
- Application problems, lack of practice.
- Some couples complain about a lack of sensitivity.
- Using oil-based lubricant with latex condoms can damage the condom.
- Expiry date has passed.

**Necessary routine**
Use a new condom for every act of intercourse.

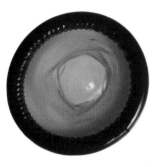

Actual Size

## WHAT IS THE CONDOM ALL ABOUT?

Condoms are sheaths made out of rubber (latex), polyurethane or animal material (sheep membrane), which are placed on the erect penis. Condoms are the only method of contraception that provide protection against pregnancy and STIs including HIV.

The cheapest and most widely used are latex condoms. People with a latex allergy can use polyurethane or sheep membrane condoms. Polyurethane condoms are as effective as latex condoms in preventing pregnancy and infection and have some unique advantages. **Sheep membrane condoms protect only against unintended pregnancy and not against STIs and HIV.** Viruses and bacteria are so small that they can pass through the pores of sheep membrane condoms. Only monogamous couples should use them.

Tactylon condoms have been introduced in the US and are not yet available in Canada.

Condoms also offer protection from infections for same sex couples. Condoms are highly recommended for sex practices such as oral and anal sex.

Since no other method of birth control (except the female condom) offers nearly full protection against infections like the latex or polyurethane condoms do, condoms should be used in combination with other methods of contraception to practice safer sex (dual protection).

In summary, the latex and polyurethane condoms protect against:
- HIV
- STIs (except HPV and Herpes)
- Pregnancy
- Ectopic pregnancy
- Lower tract infections (vaginitis)
- Upper tract infections (Pelvic Inflammatory Disease)
- Infections that can harm the fetus during pregnancy and childbearing
- Blocked fallopian tubes, which cause infertility

### How does the condom work?
Condoms act as a barrier and are protective in many ways. Latex and polyurethane condoms **protect the man** from coming into contact with secretions from the vagina, wounds inside the vagina or menstrual blood and prevent him from catching an infection.

Latex and polyurethane condoms **protect the woman** from contact with semen thus protecting her from unintended pregnancy. At the same time, the condom protects her from catching STI and HIV infections.

Sheep membrane condoms are made from the intestines of lamb. The small pores in the condom do not let semen pass but they let certain bacteria and viruses through. Sheep membrane condoms therefore only protect against pregnancy and should only be used by monogamous couples.

## How effective is the condom in preventing unintended pregnancy?

Failure is not usually due to failure of the method itself, for example a condom breaking. All condoms on the Canadian market are tested for their quality. Condoms are very effective in preventing pregnancy when used consistently and correctly. Only 2% of women who use latex condoms perfectly will become pregnant within the first year. This means that out of 100 couples who used latex condoms correctly for one year, only two couples will experience a pregnancy. The typical use failure rate is 15%. The typical use failure rate takes into account the misuse or non-use of the method. The highest failure rate is reported in women between ages 20-24.

Polyurethane condoms are as effective as latex condoms in preventing pregnancy, with the exception of eZ.on®, which has proven to be less effective.

Polyurethane condoms are fairly new on the market and not as well studied as latex condoms.

## Does the condom protect against sexually transmitted infections and HIV?

Latex condoms protect against STIs and HIV. Polyurethane condoms may be less effective due to a higher frequency of breakage and slippage shown in tests. Sheep membrane condoms do not protect against STIs and HIV.

Consistent use of condoms can reduce HIV transmission rates in the population by 85%.

**A word of caution: Latex and polyurethane condoms may not fully protect against Herpes and the Human Papilloma Virus (HPV) which causes genital warts. The reason is that these viruses are spread by skin to skin contact and found in skin areas which are not covered by the condom.**

If you are in a monogamous relationship, using a separate spermicide with a condom may be as effective as the oral contraceptive pill in preventing pregnancy. Condoms which have a spermicide built into them are not any more effective than non-spermicidal condoms.

## How popular are condoms in Canada?

In the 2002 Canadian Contraception Study, condoms were used by 21% of respondents.

## Added value: Health benefits of the condom

Condoms offer a whole lot of benefits, which make them a great method. They can be used alone or in combination with another method and they have even more to offer than just protection against pregnancy, STIs and HIV.

**A condom can improve a sexual relationship** by helping some men from ejaculating too fast. Using condoms takes practice and it can lead to better control of the time of ejaculation. This may help the woman to reach orgasm as well.

**Protection against infertility.** We know that some STIs can damage the reproductive organs and lead to infertility. By protecting against STIs, condoms also help to protect against future infertility.

**More hygienic.** The condom prevents semen from entering the vagina. The messy discharge after intercourse does not occur when using a condom.

**Protection against cervical cancer.** Cervical cancer is associated with some viruses (HIV and HPV). The condom prevents the transmission of some of these viruses. The protection offered by condoms is only partial, however.

**Not convinced yet? Think of this**

Here are more features that make condoms a great method:
- Easy to get and relatively inexpensive.
- Great variety available to make the method more fun.
- Discreet to carry.
- Possible enhancement of erection.

- Prevents development of sperm allergy in women.
- Condom can be part of sex play and both partners can participate.
- Immediate, visible proof of effectiveness.

**You are right, there are some flaws as well. Condom use...**

- requires motivation, practice and sense of responsibility
- may reduce sensitivity
- may interfere with erection
- may interrupt foreplay
- may interfere with enjoyment
- may cause embarrassment
- may give unpleasant taste

## Where do I get condoms?
Nothing is easier than buying condoms. They are available in vending machines in washrooms, in drugstores, supermarkets, convenience stores, on-line, and in condom shops.

## What condoms are available in Canada?
Latex condoms come in

- dry or lubricated form
- with spermicide or without
- plain or reservoir-tipped
- straight or shaped
- smooth or textured
- different colours
- different tastes
- different sizes (small, medium, and large).

Please note: spermicidal condoms are not more effective than non-spermicidal condoms. If you are in a monogamous relationship and want to add a spemicide you should use a separate product in addition to the condom (see section on spermicides, pages 108-113).

Choosing a polyurethane condom is easier because there are only a few brands. They are more expensive than latex condoms but sensation tends to be less affected than with latex condoms. They transmit body heat better than latex condoms, feel thinner and have a less constricting fit.

Novelty condoms, offered in sex shops, catalogues or on-line are considered sex toys and do not offer pregnancy and STI/HIV protection.

## It can be so much fun
It's a matter of trying and checking out what you and your partner prefer. Condoms are by far the most fun method of contraception because the choice of models is so great. When you and your partner become familiar and comfortable with the use of a condom you have a wealth of possibilities to choose from. Different models might help you to improve your sex life! Get started and check it out!

A word of caution: always read the package insert! Some sophisticated models, such as novelty condoms, (special taste, special colour) have undergone certain treatments that make them less protective. This is clearly marked on the pack. The quality of latex can deteriorate with certain treatments, which are indicated in the inserts. The material also deteriorates when it comes into contact with oil-based products, such as Vaseline (petroleum jelly) and vaginal medicated creams.

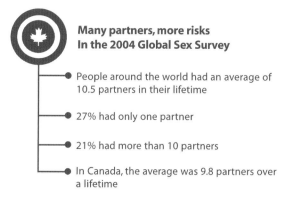

**Many partners, more risks
In the 2004 Global Sex Survey**

- People around the world had an average of 10.5 partners in their lifetime
- 27% had only one partner
- 21% had more than 10 partners
- In Canada, the average was 9.8 partners over a lifetime

# HOW DO I USE CONDOMS?

1. Check the expiry date. When condoms are expired they do not protect any more.

2. Check the package. It should be sealed and not ripped. Do not use unpackaged condoms because the exposure to light weakens them within hours.

3. Do not do any of your own testing like filling them with water or blowing a balloon to check whether they are intact! Experts have already done this! Your own testing might damage the condom!

4. Trial makes you the master. In the privacy of your bedroom, follow the instructions and apply the condom on the erect penis. Do this BEFORE you practice it with your partner. It will give you more self-assurance and will make it easier when it's time for the real thing! Try to put on the condom when it is dark or with your eyes closed as well.

5. Put a drop of water-based lubricant or saliva on the tip of the condom, which improves sensation with the condom.

6. Place the rolled condom over the tip of the erect penis.

7. Leave a centimeter space at the tip of the condom to collect the semen if the condom does not already have a reservoir at the tip.

8. If not circumcised, pull back the foreskin with one hand.

9. Pinch the air out of the tip.

10. Unroll the condom over the penis. Unroll it all the way down to the base of the penis.

11. Smooth out any air bubbles.

12. Lubricate the outside of the condom before entering the vagina.

13. Immediately after ejaculation: be careful not to spill any semen. Hold the condom on the base of the penis while pulling out of the vagina. Pull out before the penis softens!

14. Throw the condom in the trash.

15. Wash penis with water and soap before any further contact.

16. Use a new condom each time you have intercourse!

---

### TELL ME WHY

**Of the 1582 women interviewed during the 2002 Canadian Contraception Study**
- 21% used condoms as their present method.

Surprisingly, their main reasons were:
- birth control: 66%
- STI prevention: 5%
- Both: 25%

# TROUBLESHOOTING

The most common complaints with condoms are that they interfere with the sexplay and that they decrease sensitivity. All of this need not happen if you and your partner are willing to put some effort into practicing! Here are some tips:

- Include condoms in your foreplay.
- Have the partner place the condom over the partner's penis.
- Make it a "fun experiment".
- Try different models until you find the right one that suits you!

Other problems might be...

### My partner does not like to use a condom

This is a tough one...you have to convince your partner. Be creative! Here are some selling tools for you:

- One of you might have an STI without knowing or feeling anything at all.
- STIs and HIV infections can happen to anybody, no matter who you are.
- The majority of STIs are potentially more damaging to the woman than to the man. That's because many STIs infect the reproductive organs of the woman and may lead to infertility.

### Losing the erection

A woman should always be supportive if the partner has a problem with his erection. After all, the man is showing responsibility by using a condom and the woman should encourage this. Putting on the condom could be part of making love. Masturbation and oral pleasuring techniques might help.

### Condoms do not allow for spontaneity

If you and your partner make condom use a part of your sex play, there shouldn't be any problem with spontaneity.

### Condom breaks

This very rarely happens with the condoms that are available today. Condom breakage also does not necessarily lead to pregnancy. Reasons for breakage are rough handling, use of oil-based lubricant on latex condoms or expired condoms. Refer to page 84 for advice and consult for emergency contraception as soon as possible!

### Condom slips off during intercourse

It can happen when too much lubricant was used on the inside of the condom. Take it off completely and use a new one with less lubricant. Consult for emergency contraception as soon as possible!

### VERY IMPORTANT:

- Use a condom EVERY time you have sex.
- Use a NEW condom for each act of intercourse.
- Keep the condoms in a dark and dry place away from heat.
- Always have a spermicide with an applicator handy to use with the condom and to use in an emergency when the condom slips or breaks. Then go to the pharmacy for emergency contraception.
- **Use only water-based lubricants** with the latex condom. Please refer to page 84 for different lubricants.
- **Use water or oil-based lubricants with the polyurethane condom.**
- For mouth to penis contact use flavoured condoms or condoms which are dry (not pre-treated with a lubricant) to avoid bad taste.

**LUBRICANTS AND PRODUCTS THAT ARE SAFE OR UNSAFE TO USE WITH LATEX CONDOMS**

## SAFE

- Aloe-9
- Aqua-Lube
- Aqua-Lube Plus
- Astroglide
- Carbowax
- Condom-mate
- Contraceptive foams (e.g. Delfen)
- Contraceptive creams and gels (e.g. Ramses)
- Duragel
- Egg white
- Forplay lubricant, saliva
- Glycerin usp
- Intercept
- Koromex gel
- KY Jelly
- Lubafax
- Lubrin insert
- Ortho-Gynol
- Personal Lubricant
- Prepair Lubricant
- Probe
- Semicid
- Saliva
- Silicones DC 360
- Transi-Lube
- Water

## UNSAFE

- Baby oils
- Burn ointments
- Coconut oil/butter
- All oils (peanut, sunflower, olive, corn...)
- Fish oils
- Haemorrhoid ointments
- Insect repellents
- Margarine, butter
- Mineral oil
- Palm oil
- Vaseline (petroleum jelly)
- Rubbing alcohol
- Suntan oil
- Vaginal creams (Monistat, Esterase, Femstat, Vagisil, Premarin, Rendell's Cone, Pharmatex Ovule)
- Some sexual lubricants (e.g. Elbow Grease, Hot Elbow grease, Shaft)

### RECOMMENDATIONS FOR CONDOM BREAKAGE AND SLIPPAGE

➡ Immediately insert spermicidal foam or gel

➡ If no spermicidal product is available, immediately wash both penis and vagina with soap and water

➡ Consult for emergency contraception

## A WORD ABOUT SPERMICIDES

The medical community has become more cautious about recommending spermicides. Studies have shown that spermicides increase the risk for HIV infections because nonoxynol-9 may irritate the mucosa of the vagina. These studies were done with women who used spermicides more than once a day. A less frequent use of nonoxynol-9 probably does not cause any irritations.

To be on the safe side, we recommend the following:
1. Spermicides are a contraceptive for women who are at low risk for STIs and HIV, for example women in monogamous relationships in which STIs and HIV have been ruled out.
2. Methods which need an added spermicide, such as diaphragm, cervical cap and sponge should therefore only be used by monogamous couples.
3. Only latex or polyurethane condoms offer protection against STIs and HIV infections.
4. Do not use spermicides to prevent STIs and HIV. Always use a condom.
5. Use uncoated condoms, rather than nonoxynol-9 coated condoms.
6. If you only have nonoxynol-9 coated condoms you can use them because they are better than not using a condom at all!

For your own and your partner's health:
Say NO to sex if your partner says NO to condoms
NO GLOVE, NO LOVE!

# FEMALE CONDOM

**Who controls the show?**
The woman.

**What is the female condom all about?**
A polyurethane sheath with two rings inside for women to wear during vaginal intercourse. It protects against pregnancy, STIs and HIV.

**How do I get it?**
Prescription-free, in drugstores, family planning clinics or on-line.

**How do I use it?**
Insert it in the vagina before intercourse. Insertion can be done hours before intercourse.

**If you use a lubricant**
Water- or oil-based lubricants.

**How effective is the female condom in preventing unintended pregnancy?**
79-95% effective.

**Does the female condom protect against sexually transmitted infections and HIV?**
Yes.

**What makes the female condom so special?**
It is the only contraceptive controlled by women that protects against pregnancy and STI/HIV.

**Possible problems**
Insertion difficulties, sound during sex.

**Necessary routine**
Use a new condom for every act of intercourse.

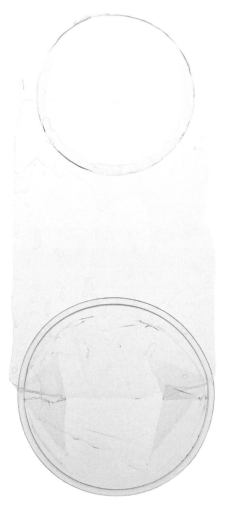

## WHAT IS THE FEMALE CONDOM ALL ABOUT?

It is a polyurethane sheath, which is a thin and supple kind of plastic. When you compare it with condoms made for man:

- It does **not** contain latex.
- It is bigger in size because it has to fit the size of the vagina.
- It has two rings. The inner ring at the closed end of the condom is used to insert the condom and to keep it in place. It slides in place behind the pubic bone, acting like an anchor for the condom. The outer ring remains outside the vagina and partially covers and protects the lips of the vagina.

There is only one brand available in Canada, which is called Reality Female Condom®.

**It is the only method controlled by the woman that provides dual protection: it protects against unintended pregnancy and STIs and HIV.**

### How does it work?

The woman places the female condom into her vagina before intercourse, or more precisely, before any vaginal contact with the partner. The condom fits against the walls of the vagina and has a double effect:

1. It prevents the semen from getting into the vagina.
2. It prevents the exchange of body fluids between both partners.

The outer ring of the condom protects the lips at the entrance of the vagina. The female condom offers protection against unintended pregnancy, sexually transmitted infections and HIV.

**Can the condom disappear inside the vagina?**

The outer ring holds it in place even if movements become very intense during intercourse. The condom can be removed easily after intercourse by pulling with two fingers. However, if it disappears you have to interrupt lovemaking and put it back in place.

? **Can I pass urine while the condom is in place?**

No problem. The urine passes through a different canal than the vagina. It is called the urethra, which is above the vagina under the pubic bone. You can interrupt lovemaking at any time to go to the washroom, leaving the condom in place.

# SPECIAL FEATURES OF THE FEMALE CONDOM

The female condom was introduced in Canada in 1996. What is true for many things is especially true for the female condom: you won't know if you'll like it unless you really try it! Here are some features of the condom that might spark your interest:

- Your male partner does not like to use a condom because of a latex allergy or because of general dislike; the female condom is an excellent alternative.

- People with a latex allergy can use the female condom because it is made out of polyurethane.

- The condom is made out of a very thin plastic, which warms up instantly to body temperature. It is thinner than the usual male condoms and allows for a more natural feeling and sensitivity during lovemaking.

- The condom has a lubricant on the outside and inside. The outside lubricant combines with the natural lubrication in the vagina and makes the condom fit against the walls of the vagina. The inside lubricant helps the penis to enter the condom.

- Unlike the condom worn by the male, the female condom is spacious and does not fit tightly on the penis. This is a great advantage considering that some men don't like to use condoms because they feel they are too tight on their penis.

- To make the entry of the penis into the vagina easier you can use water, or oil-based lubricants or moisturizers. There are sachets of extra lubricant, which come with the female condom in the same pack.

- The condom can be inserted 8 hours before intercourse, meaning you do not have to interrupt lovemaking. This is a great advantage considering that the condom used by the male partner can only be put on during sex when the penis is erect.

- After intercourse you can take your time before removing the condom. It does not have to be done immediately afterwards but before standing up.

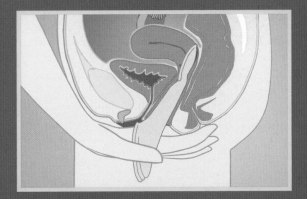

# HOW DO I USE THE FEMALE CONDOM?

**(1)** Study the package insert. It sounds like a boring idea but... the package insert contains illustrations and very good explanations.

**(2)** Trial makes you the master. Use one condom and insert it as directed. In the heat of the moment when you are planning to have intercourse you do not want to stop and read the instructions first.

**(3)** Talk to your partner about trying it.

**Let's talk about it!**
It is a good idea to tell your partner about this method before you use it for the first time with him. This way you can prepare him, and you will not have any discussion in the middle of lovemaking! If your partner normally uses a condom you will have to tell him that he cannot use it when you use the female condom. Two condoms together do not work!

**Here are some important things to remember:**

➡ Use the female condom every time you have sex.

➡ Use a new condom with each sex act. After ejaculation you have to remove the condom BEFORE standing up and throw it in the garbage. (Not into the toilet because it might block it!)

➡ Guide the penis into the outer ring to make sure that it does not go on the side, passing the condom by.

➡ A good lubrication inside the condom is important for a smooth ride! Use more lubricant if the penis sticks to the condom and cannot move freely. You can even use lotion or other oil-based products if you do not have water-based lubricants with you.

## How effective is the female condom in preventing unintended pregnancy?

When used properly and consistently it is as effective as the male condom. Statistically speaking, only 5 out of 100 women using the female condom correctly over a period of one year may become pregnant. The failure rate for typical use over a 12-month-period is 21%.

## Does the female condom protect against sexually transmitted infections and HIV?

YES. This is the only contraceptive controlled by the female that protects against sexually transmitted infections and HIV.

## How popular is the female condom in Canada?

In the 2002 Canadian Contraception Study, the female condom was used by 1% of respondents.

## Where do I get the female condom?

In the drugstore or on-line. You do not need a prescription.

**FREQUENCY OF SEX AND ORGASMS
From the 2004 Global Sex Survey we found out that**

- Canadians have sex on average 108 times per year (global average of the 41 countries in the survey is 103 times)

- 36% have orgasms every time they have sex (global average is 35%)

# TROUBLESHOOTING

**The most common complaint with the female condom is difficulty with the insertion (that's why we highly recommend that you practice!). Others might be...**

### The condom makes noise

Obviously it cannot make noise on its own...it depends on the action! Relax! This can even be fun. The noise depends on the shape of the vagina, which is responsible for the fit of the female condom. It also depends on the movement of the penis in the vagina. You can always try the following to change the noise: change the position during lovemaking. You may also want to add more lubricant on the partner's penis.

### The condom breaks

This is very unlikely because the material the female condom is made of is about 40% stronger than the latex condom. If you are in a monogamous relationship use an applicator and apply spermicide into the vagina immediately. In any case, refer to Chapter 8 on emergency contraception.

**IN A NUTSHELL**

# CONTRACEPTIVE SPONGE

### Who controls the show?
The woman.

### What is the sponge all about?
A disposable barrier made out of polyurethane foam, which is placed at the cervix. It absorbs and traps sperm. For additional protection the sponge contains spermicides that destroy sperm. Should only be used in monogamous relationships.

### How do I get it?
Prescription-free, in drugstores, family planning clinics, on-line.

### How do I use it?
Insert it into the vagina in front of the cervix at least 15 minutes before intercourse.

### How effective is the sponge in preventing unintended pregnancy?
- 68-80% effective in parous women (those who have already given birth).
- 84-91% effective in nulliparous women (women who have not given birth).

### Does the sponge protect against sexually transmitted infections and HIV?
The spermicides in the sponge provide protection against some STIs, but not HIV.

### What makes the sponge so special?
- It is a barrier method and a spermicide in one product.
- 12-hour protection against pregnancy.
- No change of sponge necessary if intercourse is repeated within the 12-hour period.

### Possible problems
- Difficulties in removing the sponge.
- Forgetting to take out the sponge because you forget all about it.
- Allergy against the foam or the spermicides.
- Vaginal irritations which increase the risk of HIV transmission.

### Necessary routine
Never reinsert a used sponge.

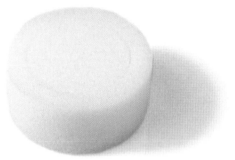

Actual Size

## WHAT IS THE CONTRACEPTIVE SPONGE ALL ABOUT?

It is a disposable, one-size-fits-all polyurethane foam device that fits over the cervix. The sponge is round and has two slots for the fingers to fit in to make insertion and removal easy. There are two products available in Canada, Protectaid® and Today®.

### How does the contraceptive sponge work?
It is inserted into the vagina to cover the entrance of the uterus (cervix). The sponge does two things:
1. It acts as a barrier to prevent the sperm from entering the cervix by absorbing and trapping sperm.
2. The Protectaid® sponge contains F-5 Gel, a combination of spermicides that destroy sperm. The spermicides are nonoxynol-9, benzalkonium chloride and sodium cholate. The Today® sponge contains nonoxynol-9.

The concentrations of spermicides are low, reducing the possibility of irritation in the vaginal wall and on the penis. The sponge provides protection for 12 hours.

### How effective is the sponge in preventing unintended pregnancy?
Sponges are more effective in women who have not given birth (nulliparous) as compared to women who have given birth (parous). After one year of typical use of Protectaid®, 16% of nulliparous women and 32% of parous women became pregnant, while 20% of nulliparous and 40% of parous women became pregnant with Today®.

When the sponge is used in combination with the male condom the efficacy rises to a failure rate of only 2%.

### Does the sponge protect against sexually transmitted infections and HIV?
The sponge when used alone does not sufficiently protect against STIs and HIV. The sponge should be used in combination with a male latex condom.

There is some evidence that the spermicide in the sponge changes the mucosa of the vagina, leading to irritations, which can actually increase the risk of HIV infections. This is the reason why sponges should only be used in monogamous relationships in which there is no risk of HIV infection. Practice safer sex: use a condom for dual protection!

### How popular is the sponge in Canada?
The 2002 Canadian Contraception study showed that sponges were used by less than 1% of respondents.

### Where do I get the sponge?
Prescription-free, in the drugstore, in a family planning clinic or on-line.

---

### IMPORTANT POINTS TO KEEP IN MIND:
- Use a new sponge every time you have sex
- Never reuse a sponge
- Practice! Insertion needs some practice
- Do not use during menstruation
- Do not forget to take it out! It may be forgotten and left in place because it cannot be felt: potential risk for Toxic Shock Syndrome

## HOW DO I USE THE SPONGE?

1. Check expiry date
2. Read the package insert
3. Practice the insertion for yourself

➡ Wash hands with soap before touching sponge and inserting it

➡ Keep timing in mind: insert at least 15 minutes before intercourse; take it out at the earliest 6 hours after intercourse

➡ Do not use a vaginal douche with the sponge in place

➡ Throw the used sponge in the trash

➡ NEVER reinsert a used sponge

## SPECIAL FEATURES OF THE SPONGE

**Timing:**

- Sponge can be inserted hours before intercourse.
- Insert sponge at least 15 minutes before lovemaking.
- Sponge provides continuous protection for 12 hours.
- No new sponge needed if another act of intercourse happens within 12 hours.
- After intercourse: leave the sponge in place for a minimum of 6 hours.
- But: the sponge should not stay in the vagina longer than 12 hours.

**Action:**

- Sponge has a double action (spermicide to destroy sperm and barrier against sperm).
- No systemic reactions.

**Convenience:**

- Easy to carry.
- Prescription-free.
- No fitting, no physician required.
- Insertion does not interrupt sex play.
- Sponge cannot be felt by either partner.
- No leakage of semen through the vagina after ejaculation because the sponge absorbs semen.

# TROUBLESHOOTING

**The following problems might occur and they could be a signal to you to make an appointment with your physician.**

### Odour ⚠

If there is an unpleasant smell after removing the sponge, do not be concerned. Any material placed in the vagina that comes into contact with vaginal fluids and possibly semen will catch a smell. However, if the sponge has a different colour than before and the smell from the vagina stays even for days after removal of the sponge, you should make an appointment with a healthcare professional.

### Yeast infection/Bacterial vaginosis ⚠

Some sponge users have a problem with recurrent yeast infections and bacterial vaginosis. You should ask your physician whether you should consider another method of contraception. However, clinical studies with Protectaid® did not show any increased incidence of infections with long-term use.

### Allergy against spermicides or polyurethane ⚠

If you develop an allergic reaction to any of the ingredients that make up a sponge you will have to consider another method.

### Toxic shock syndrome (TSS) ⚠

This is a very serious and very rare medical condition that you might have heard about in reference to tampon use during menstruation. If the sponge has been left in for a prolonged time and if you experience two or more of the warning signals you have to go to the emergency room of a hospital immediately:

- sudden high fever
- diarrhoea
- vomiting
- dizziness
- weakness
- muscle aches, sunburn-like rash in the palms of the hands or on the soles of the feet

**IN A NUTSHELL**

# DIAPHRAGM

**Who controls the show?**
The woman.

**What is the diaphragm all about?**
A flat latex or silicon cap with an enclosed ring, which fits against the entrance of the cervix. It holds spermicide over the cervical opening. The diaphragm must be used in combination with a spermicide (gel or cream) to ensure protection. The spermicide destroys the sperm. Should only be used in monogamous relationships.

**How do I get it?**
You need an appointment with your family physician, gynaecologist or family planning clinic to get a diaphragm fitted for your body.

**How do I use it?**
Insert the diaphragm by hand through the vagina in front of the cervix anytime before intercourse.

**If you use a lubricant**
Only water-based products for latex diaphragms.

**Does the diaphragm protect against sexually transmitted infections and HIV?**
NO. The diaphragm with the spermicide added to it by the user protects against bacterial infections. The protection against viral infections has not been proven. Spermicides may cause vaginal irritation which increases the risk of HIV transmission.

**How effective is the diaphragm in preventing unintended pregnancy?**
84-94% effective.

**What makes the diaphragm so special?**
- A very private method because the diaphragm can be inserted up to 6 hours before intercourse.
- The insertion needs some practice and a motivated user.
- It has to be used with a spermicide.

**What makes it different from the cervical cap?**
- It is bigger.
- It is easier to insert.
- It needs more spermicide.
- You have to apply more spermicide for each repeated act of intercourse.
- Higher risk of urinary tract infections.
- Can be used during menstruation.

**Possible problems**
- Women suffering from urinary tract infections should not use it. There is a possibility of developing UTI while using the diaphragm.
- Insertion problems.
- Wrong fit.
- Vaginal irritation which increase the risk of HIV transmission.

**Necessary routine**
Apply new spermicide and insert diaphragm every time you have sex.

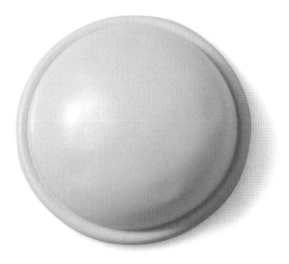

## WHAT IS THE DIAPHRAGM ALL ABOUT?

A diaphragm is a cap (made from latex or silicon), which covers the cervix and a part of the vagina. It has a flexible steel ring on the edge to help keep its shape. The steel ring is surrounded by soft material and cannot cause any harm. **This barrier method must be used in combination with a spermicide (gel or cream) to give sufficient protection against unintended pregnancy.**

### How does the diaphragm work?

The woman has to place the diaphragm through the vagina around the cervix up to 6 hours before intercourse. There the diaphragm and spermicide destroy the sperm and prevent sperm from getting into the cervix. During intercourse the vagina is moving and the diaphragm is not always a perfect seal on the cervix. This is why the diaphragm has to be used with a spermicide to increase protection against pregnancy.

### How effective is the diaphragm in preventing unintended pregnancy?

If used perfectly (meaning it fits you well and you use it every time you have sex) the failure rate during the first year of use is 6%. In other words: of 100 women who used the diaphragm consistently and correctly during a one-year study, 6 became pregnant. The failure rate for 12 month of typical use is 16%.

### Does the diaphragm protect against sexually transmitted infections and HIV?

It does not fully protect because there is still an exchange of body fluids (semen and natural lubrication of the vagina) between partners. However, there is a reduced risk of bacterial infection due to the fact that semen does not enter the cervix. The spermicide protects against STIs caused by bacteria, however, **protection against viral infections has not been proven.** In fact, spermicide use may cause vaginal irritation and increase the risk of HIV transmission. The male partner should use a latex condom to protect both partners from a possible infection. Practice safer sex: use dual protection!

### Where do I get a diaphragm?

You have to make an appointment with your family physician, gynaecologist or family planning clinic. A pelvic exam and a medical history will be taken. For more information on the pelvic exam refer to Chapter 3.

The pelvic exam is necessary to fit you with the right type and size of diaphragm. The size and type will depend upon your build and whether or not you have had children. Therefore it is not a good idea to obtain a diaphragm through an on-line pharmacy and try to fit it yourself. The physician will explain to you how to insert it and will let you insert it yourself in the changing room.

Afterwards he/she will check whether it fits well and if you have inserted it correctly. The sure sign that it fits well is that you do not feel it at all. With the prescription you can buy the diaphragm at the pharmacy and use it for years when you take care of it properly.

### Storage and care

Wash it with warm water and mild soap, rinse it, dry it and put it back in the box. Keep it away from light and excessive heat. Keep the storage box in a place where you will find it afterwards (with your toothbrush for example). The empty box will remind you to take the diaphragm out and will save you from forgetting! Replace it when it is damaged or bent. It is good for a year or two if you look after it well!

### What types of diaphragms are available in Canada?

There are 2 different types available in Canada. They are made from latex and they are offered in various sizes. A silicon diaphragm can be ordered on the Internet (wide-seal).

### How popular is the diaphragm in Canada?

No data available.

## SPECIAL FEATURES OF THE DIAPHRAGM

Here are some facts that make it an interesting alternative to other methods:

**Timing:**

You can insert the diaphragm up to 6 hours before intercourse. This is an advantage because you do not have to bother about it when you are in the middle of lovemaking.

It has to be left inside the vagina for a minimum of 6 hours after intercourse. The diaphragm should not be worn longer than 24 hours because serious infections can occur.

**Action:**

You have to use a spermicide with the diaphragm. For each repeated act of intercourse you will have to use additional spermicide using an applicator while leaving the device in place.

**Caution:**

If you or your partner has a problem with latex products you should not use a latex diaphragm.

**Be motivated:**

You have to carry your diaphragm with you and you always have to have spermicidal gel or cream with an applicator handy!

# HOW DO I USE A DIAPHRAGM?

**1** Study the package insert. It sounds like a boring idea but... the package insert contains helpful illustrations and very good explanations.

**2** Trial makes you the master. Insert it as directed. In the heat of the moment when you are planning to have intercourse you do not want to stop the action, read the instructions and get all nervous.

**3** Walk around with the diaphragm in place. Do some exercise and make sure you do not feel it. If you do feel it even when it is placed correctly you will have to contact your physician and get it exchanged.

**4** Take it out, wash it and try it again. For the removal: Insert a finger in the vagina, locate the rim of the diaphragm. Hook the finger behind it and pull it out.

**5** Better be safe than sorry. The first few times you use the diaphragm your partner should use a condom until you are sure you get it right!

**6** If you need dual protection, ask your partner to use a condom.

**Avoid common mistakes and do the following:**

→ Use the diaphragm EVERY time you have sex, also during your period.

→ Wash your hands before touching and inserting the diaphragm.

→ Hold it against the light to check for holes and tears. If there is any damage it does not protect you.

→ Check expiry date of spermicide.

→ Apply a spermicide in the cup of the diaphragm.

→ Insert the diaphragm with spermicide inside (you know how, practiced before, right?).

→ Apply more spermicide after each act of intercourse without taking the diaphragm out. You need a spermicide with an applicator to reach into the vagina for that.

→ If you want to use a lubricant or moisturizer, use only water-based lubricants or moisturizers with the latex diaphragm.

→ Wait 6-8 hours after intercourse to take it out. You do not have to set an alarm clock for this but it should not be in your vagina longer than 24 hours.

→ Do not use a vaginal douche.

# TROUBLESHOOTING

### Difficulty with insertion ⚠

The most common complaint with the diaphragm is difficulty with the insertion (that's why we highly recommend that you practice!). One major mistake: too much spermicide! If the spermicide is all over the diaphragm it will become too slippery to handle when you fold it for insertion. The solution is: use only 1-2 teaspoons of spermicide in the cup of the diaphragm (depends on size of the diaphragm) and PRACTICE!

### Refitting necessary when... ⚠

You might need another size of diaphragm after giving birth, after an abortion, after surgery in the pelvis or if you experienced a big loss or increase in body weight. You have to make an appointment with your physician.

### Diaphragm goes out of place during lovemaking ⚠

In this case sperm from the pre-ejaculate or the ejaculate may have passed the barrier. Apply some more spermicide immediately. Contact your local pharmacy for emergency contraception.

### Urinary tract infections (UTI) ⚠

Diaphragms can increase the risk of urinary tract infections due to the pressure of the flexible steel ring on the urethra. If you suffer from UTI (infections in the bladder or urethra that make it painful to pass urine) it is better not to use the diaphragm as a method of contraception. If you develop UTI while using the diaphragm, your physician might prescribe another type for you (with another rim that puts less pressure on the urethra).

### Toxic shock syndrome (TSS) ⚠

Do not leave the diaphragm in the vagina for longer than 24 hours. For TSS danger signs go to page 95.

**IN A NUTSHELL**

# CERVICAL CAP

### Who controls the show?
The woman.

### What is the cervical cap all about?
A deep silicon cap that fits against the entrance of the cervix. It prevents sperm and bacteria from entering the cervix. The cervical cap must be used with spermicidal cream or gel. The spermicide destroys sperm. Should only be used in monogamous relationships.

### How do I get it?
You need an appointment at a clinic or with your gynaecologist who will examine you to find out the correct size of cervical cap to fit you perfectly. You will get a prescription to buy the cap at a pharmacy, clinic or on-line.

### How do I use it?
Insert it through the vagina in front of the cervix anytime before intercourse.

### If you use a lubricant
Water- or oil-based products.

### How effective is the cervical cap in preventing unintended pregnancy?
- 68-74% effective in parous women (women who have given birth).
- 84-91% effective in nulliparous women (those who have not given birth).

### Does the cervical cap protect against sexually transmitted infections and HIV?
NO. The cervical cap with the spermicide added to it by the user protects against bacterial infections. The protection against viral infections has not been proven. Spermicides may cause vaginal irritation which increases the risk of HIV transmission.

### What makes the cervical cap so special?
- A very private method, does not interfere with love-making because it can be inserted before.
- Insertion needs some practice and requires a motivated user.
- It has to be used with a spermicide.

### What makes it different from the diaphragm?
- It is smaller.
- Insertion might need more practice.
- Requires less spermicide.
- Lower risk of urinary tract infections.
- **Must not be used during menstruation.**

### Possible problems
- A sensitivity or allergy towards rubber or spermicide is a reason not to use it.
- The annual PAP smear is important to check possible inflammation in cervix.
- Insertion problems.
- Wrong fit.
- Dislodgement during intercourse.
- Vaginal irritation which increase the risk of HIV.

### Necessary routine
Apply new spermicide and reinsert cervical cap every time you have sex.

by suction. During intercourse the vagina is moving and the cap is not always a perfect seal on the cervix. For better protection the cervical cap has to be used with spermicidal cream or gel in and around the cap.

### How effective is the cap in preventing unintended pregnancy?

There is a difference in effectiveness when used by women who have already given birth (parous) and women who have not (nulliparous). If used perfectly, (meaning it fits you well and you insert the cap correctly every time you have sex) the failure rate during the first year of use is 9% in nulliparous women. This means that over a one-year study, 9 pregnancies occurred in 100 couples who used the cervical cap.

If used perfectly, the failure rate during the first year of use in parous women is 26%.

Studies have shown a much higher failure rate in the first year of typical use among nulliparous (16%) and parous women (32%). The use of spermicidal cream or gel is very important to insure better protection against pregnancy.

The effectiveness of the cervical cap depends on the correct fit over the cervix and on the correct insertion by the woman. That's where your skills come in! Any event that might change the shape of the cervix (birth, abortion, weight change of +/- 3 kg, and other surgery) makes a refitting of the cervical cap necessary.

### Does the cap protect against sexually transmitted infections and HIV?

The cervical cap protects the ovaries and the uterus from sperm and bacteria.

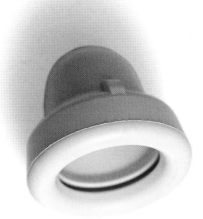

Actual Size

## WHAT IS THE CERVICAL CAP ALL ABOUT?

A cervical cap is a small silicon cap with a flexible ring around the edge. It fits over the entrance of the cervix to prevent sperm from entering the uterus. **This barrier method has to be used in combination with a spermicide applied before insertion of the cap (gel or cream) to give sufficient protection against unintended pregnancy.**

### How does the cervical cap work?

The woman has to push the cervical cap through the vagina and place it over the cervix. There the cervical cap acts like a barrier in front of the cervix and prevents semen from entering the cervix. It is smaller than a diaphragm and it is held in place

The vagina and the penis are still exposed to body fluids such as sperm and the natural lubrication of the vagina. To summarize:

- **There is a reduced risk of bacterial infection** due to the fact that sperm does not enter the cervix and because of the protective effect of the spermicide.
- **Protection against viral infections has not been proven**. Spermicide use may cause vaginal irritation and increases the risk of HIV transmission. The male partner should use a condom to protect both partners from a possible infection.

Practice safer sex: use dual protection!

### How popular is the cervical cap in Canada?
No data available.

### Where do I get a cervical cap?
You have to make an appointment with your family physician, gynaecologist or family planning clinic. Avoid the following time periods during which the fitting of the cap cannot be done:

- Within 6 weeks after giving birth.
- Within 6 weeks of an abortion or other pelvic surgery.
- During menstruation.

A pelvic exam and a medical history will be taken. For more information about the pelvic exam refer to chapter 3. A Pap smear will be performed to rule out any infections. The pelvic exam is necessary to fit you with the right size of cervical cap. The size and type will depend upon your build and whether or not you have had children. The cap has to fit your cervix. After insertion it is kept in place by suction and for best protection it is important that it fits well.

Your healthcare professional will explain to you how to insert it and will let you insert it yourself in the changing room. Afterwards he/she will check whether it fits well and if you've inserted it correctly. The sure sign that it fits well is that it adheres to the cervix like a suction disk. With the prescription you can buy the cervical cap at the pharmacy and use it for at least a year.

A follow-up visit with your physician after 3 months is a good idea to check whether the method fits your lifestyle and to solve any problems you might have with it.

### Storage and care
Wash it with warm water and mild soap, rinse it, dry it with a cloth and put it back in the box. Keep it away from light and excessive heat.

Keep the storage box in a place where you will find it afterwards (with your toothbrush for example). The empty box will remind you to take the cervical cap out and will save you from forgetting!

Replace it when it is damaged. With proper care it can last for years.

### What types of cervical caps are available in Canada?
There is one type available: Ovès®.

## SPECIAL FEATURES OF THE CERVICAL CAP

Here are some facts that make it an interesting alternative to other methods:

**Timing:**

You can insert the cap hours before intercourse. This is an advantage because you do not have to bother about it when you are in the middle of "things"...After intercourse you can leave it inserted up to 72 hours.

**Action:**

Spermicidal gel or cream is a must.

You have to use a spermicide with the cap at the time of insertion. For each repeated act of intercourse you should use additional spermicide while leaving the device in place. You need to have spermicidal cream or gel in an applicator to insert it into the vagina.

**Caution:**

If you just gave birth, had an abortion or other pelvic surgery, the cervical cap is not for you.

**Be motivated:**

You have to carry your cervical cap with you and you always have to have spermicidal cream or gel handy!

# HOW DO I USE THE CERVICAL CAP?

**1** Study the package insert. It sounds like a boring idea but...the package insert contains illustrations and very good explanations.

**2** Trial makes you the master. Insert it as directed. In the heat of the moment when you are planning to have intercourse you do not want to stop the action, read the instructions and get all nervous.

**3** Walk around with the cervical cap in place. Do some exercise and make sure you do not feel it. If you feel it you will have to try again or see your physician to fit you with another size of cap.

**4** Take it out, wash it and try it again. For removal: Insert a finger in the vagina, locate the cap rim, press on the rim until the seal against the cervix breaks and tilt it so it comes off the cervix. With the finger behind the rim, pull it out.

**5** Better to be safe than sorry: Until you are really familiar and comfortable with the insertion of the cap, you should make your partner use a condom.

**6** If you need dual protection, ask your partner to use a condom.

**Avoid common mistakes and do the following:**

➡ Use the cervical cap EVERY time you have sex. If it sits in your drawer it cannot do its job!

➡ Use another method during menstruation. <u>Do not use the cap during menstruation.</u>

➡ Wash hands before touching and inserting the cap.

➡ Hold it against the light to check for holes and tears. If there is any damage it will not protect you.

➡ Check expiry date of spermicide.

➡ Apply spermicidal cream or gel before insertion; don't fill more than 1/3 of the cap.

➡ If necessary: use lubricants or moisturizers.

➡ Insert it before intercourse so that a good seal around the cervix can develop.

➡ Wait 6-8 hours after intercourse to take it out. You do not have to set an alarm clock for this but it should not be in your vagina longer than 72 hours.

➡ Vaginal douche: not before 6 hours after the last act of intercourse.

# TROUBLESHOOTING

## Insertion problems

The most common complaint is difficulty with the insertion and expulsion. That's why we highly recommend that you practice! One major mistake is the use of too much spermicide! If you fill more than 1/3 of the cap it will become too slippery to handle.

## Foul smell and discharge

This might occur when you leave the cervical cap in place too long. Get into the habit of putting the storage box close to your toothbrush so you will remember when you brush your teeth that you still have the cap in your body. Leave it in place at least 6 hours after the last act of intercourse, but in total it shouldn't be left in place longer than 72 hours.

**A trick:** You can leave the cap in a water/chlorophyll solution for a few hours to get rid of a bad smell.

## Cervical cap goes out of place during the act of lovemaking

In this case sperm from the pre-ejaculate or the ejaculate may have passed the barrier. Apply more spermicide with an applicator immediately. Contact your local pharmacy for emergency contraception.

## Toxic shock syndrome (TSS)

Do not leave the cervical cap in the vagina for longer than 3 days. For TSS danger signs go to page 95.

# SPERMICIDES

**Who controls the show?**
The woman.

**What are spermicides all about?**
A chemical called nonoxynol-9, which comes in the form of cream, gel, foam, film or suppository. After insertion into the vagina in front of the cervix, it destroys sperm on contact.

Spermicides should be used in combination with other methods, such as the condom. Spermicides should only be used in monogamous relationships.

**How do I get spermicides?**
In the drug-store or on-line.

**How do I use them?**
Apply deep into the vagina before intercourse. When to apply before intercourse depends on the product.

**How effective are spermicides in preventing unintended pregnancy?**
71-82% effective when used alone. It becomes a very effective method when used with a barrier method.

**Do spermicides protect against sexually transmitted infections and HIV?**
Spermicides protect against some bacterial infections. On the other hand, spermicides can cause vaginal irritation, which increases the risk of HIV transmission.

This is the reason why spermicides should only be used in monogamous relationships.

**What makes spermicides so special?**
- There are many different brands available.
- It is a very effective method of contraception when used in combination with a barrier method such as the diaphragm, cervical cap and condom.
- It offers protection against bacterial infections and pelvic inflammatory disease.
- It can be used as an emergency method after an "accident" with the condom, the diaphragm or the cap.
- It lubricates the vagina and makes penetration easier.

**Possible problems**
- Irritation of entrance of vagina or tip of penis is possible.
- The timing of the application.
- Sometimes messy.

**Necessary routine**
Apply new spermicide for every act of intercourse.

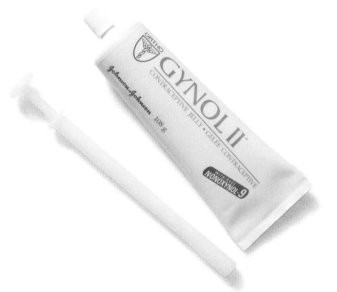

## WHAT ARE SPERMICIDES ALL ABOUT?

Spermicides are chemicals that destroy sperm and are available in the form of cream, tablet, gel, film, foam or suppository. The chemical agent used for spermicides is nonoxynol-9. They can be used alone or together with the female condom, male condom, diaphragm, and cervical cap to increase protection against pregnancy. In an emergency situation (e.g. condom slips) spermicides can also be useful.

### How do spermicides work?
Just before intercourse the woman applies spermicide in her vagina. The creams, gels or foams come with an applicator that helps to insert the substance deep into the vagina in front of the uterus. The male partner can also put spermicide directly on the condom. In fact, some condom brands already have spermicide on them. When sperm meets spermicide, a chemical reaction takes place that destroys the sperm.

### How effective are spermicides in preventing unintended pregnancy?
The consistent use of spermicides is the most important factor in minimizing failure! The failure rates of spermicides used alone range from 18% (perfect use) to 29% (typical use). The failure rate is lower when used by women who have a reduced fertility (e.g. over age 45). It is a very effective method of contraception when it is used in combination with either a cervical cap, a diaphragm, male or female condom.

If spermicides are used with another barrier method, the protection against pregnancy is comparable to hormonal methods.

### Do spermicides protect against sexually transmitted infections and HIV?
No, in fact, the use of spermicides increases the risk for HIV infections because nonoxynol-9 irritates the mucosa of the vagina. Only latex or polyurethane condoms offer protection against STI and HIV infections.

Spermicides do not seem to protect against STIs caused by bacterial infections such as chlamydia and gonorrhea. According to the World Health Organization (WHO), spermicides should not be used to prevent STIs and HIV. Always use a condom. Spermicides are a contraceptive for women who are at low risk for STI and HIV: women in monogamous relationships in which STIs and HIV have been ruled out.

### How popular are spermicides in Canada?
In the 2002 Canadian Contraception Study, spermicides were used by 1% of respondents.

**SPERMICIDES: TYPES AND TIMING**

| Product | Effective how soon after insertion | Effective for how long | Comments |
|---|---|---|---|
| FOAM | Immediately | 1 hour | Apply more spermicide for each act of intercourse |
| GEL OR CREAM | Immediately | 1 hour (if used with diaphragm or cap, 6-8 hours) | Good to use with diaphragm and cap apply more spermicide for each act of intercourse |
| FILM | 15 minutes | 1 hour | Apply more spermicide for each act of intercourse |
| SUPPOSITORY | 10-15 minutes | 1 hour | Apply more spermicide for each act of intercourse |
| BIOADHESIVE GEL ADVANTAGE 24® | Immediately | 24 hours | Apply more spermicide for each act of intercourse |

## Added value: health benefits of spermicides

Spermicides offer certain benefits apart from contraception, which should spark your interest in trying:

- Spermicides lubricate the vagina which makes intercourse smoother (if the woman lacks lubrication in the vagina). If the partner uses a condom it is also less likely to break because of the lubrication.
- Spermicides can be used in the following emergency situations to reduce the risk of becoming pregnant:
  - dislocation of cervical cap or diaphragm during intercourse.
  - breakage or leakage of condom.
- The woman can use them without the cooperation of her male partner. Unfortunately many women have difficulty convincing their partner to use condoms. With the use of spermicides the woman can have at least some protection against pregnancy.

## Where do I get spermicides?

Without a prescription in drugstores, or for more privacy, on-line.

## What spermicides are available in Canada?

Many different brands. Please refer to page 110 to get an idea of the different types of spermicides.

---

### THE DIFFERENCES BETWEEN CREAM, JELLY, FOAM, SUPPOSITORY AND FILM.

There are a variety of products available. The differences between the products are good to know to make the right choice. You have to keep two things in mind:

1. Timing: when to apply the spermicide
2. What other barrier method is being used

Some products are effective immediately when you apply them, others need some time to become effective. This can interfere with you and your partner's way of lovemaking. Page 110 gives you a summary of the various types of products.

---

You also have to read the package insert of the other barrier method you are using in combination with the spermicide. If you use a diaphragm or a cervical cap, for example, you have to buy cream or gel. For the diaphragm you need a spermicide that comes with an applicator.

The film and the foam work as well but they are not recommended with these methods. Condoms can be used with all spermicides.

# HOW DO I USE SPERMICIDES?

1. Study the package insert. It sounds like a boring idea but...the package insert contains good explanations. In this book we are only addressing the facts that apply to all spermicides on the market. But depending on which one you choose, you have to study the package insert for special instructions.

2. Trial makes you the master. For women: Insert it as directed. For men: Put some on top of your penis. This is to find out whether you are showing any allergic reactions.

3. Wait for the reaction. If you feel any irritation at the entrance of the vagina or on top of the penis, you might be allergic to the chemical and you will have to consider another method. But do not be too impatient. The feeling of irritation might disappear shortly and you are on your way!

**Common mistakes and how to avoid them: Correct placement and correct timing are important!**

➡ Use spermicide EVERY time you have sex

➡ Insert it high into the vagina following package instructions

➡ Use the required amount (no less, no more, otherwise it becomes messy)

➡ Wait the time indicated until it becomes effective before starting lovemaking

➡ Apply a new dose for every new act of intercourse

➡ Do not use a vaginal douche afterwards (wait at least 6 hours)

➡ Always have a supply handy! For foam, cream and gel you also need an applicator. When you use foam, always have an extra container handy because you might not realize when a container is running low.

➡ If applicator is used: wash it with water and soap and store it after use.

## A WORD ABOUT CONDOMS AND SPERMICIDES.

Studies have shown that the protection against pregnancy is better when condoms are used together with an extra spermicide. Some condoms are pre-treated by the manufacturer (they have a spermicide on them already) but this is less effective.

In fact, the use of spermicide-coated condoms increases the risk of urinary tract infections.

The bio-adhesive gel, Advantage 24®, has some special features that make it a spermicide easy to handle:
- Disposable applicator with the right dose: You have the right dose ready and you do not have to reuse the applicator.
- It gives 24-hour protection: you can apply the spermicide long before lovemaking, which gives you more privacy (for the very active among you: for each repeated act of intercourse you have to apply a new dose!).
- Lower concentration of nonoxynol-9 leads to fewer irritations as compared to other spermicides.
- It has a lubricant built into it as well.

# TROUBLESHOOTING

**The most common complaint with spermicides is a burning sensation or an irritation on the woman's vulva or the man's penis.**

**Other problems might be...**

### Unpleasant odour or taste

Just try different brands to find the one you and your partner like!

### Messy

Suppositories, film and Advantage 24® are less messy. Use those.

### Problem with the timing

If you dislike waiting until the spermicide is effective, use foam, gel or cream because they are effective immediately after insertion. Have a look at the table for a comparison. The new bioadhesive gel Advantage 24® can even be inserted over 20 hours before intercourse.

### Allergy

If you feel an allergic reaction when applying the spermicide you might be allergic to nonoxynol-9 (the spermicidal agent) or some other ingredient which is in the product. Try another product with different ingredients. They are marked on the package.

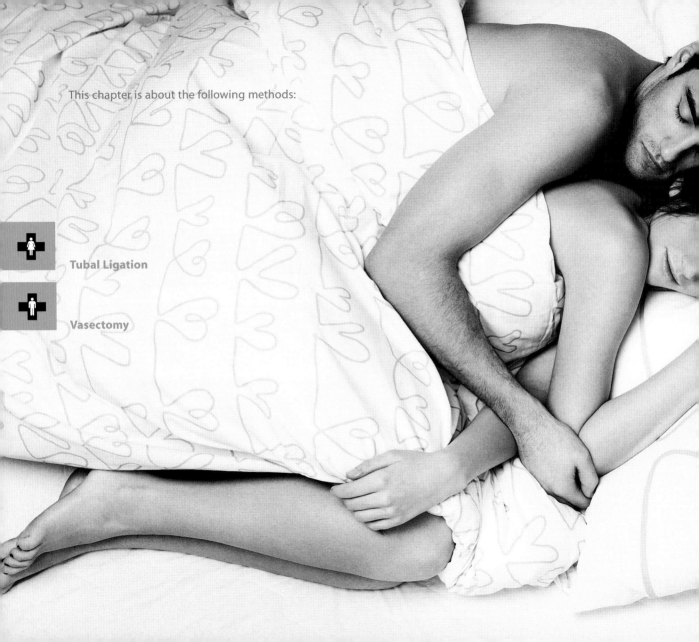

This chapter is about the following methods:

**Tubal Ligation**

**Vasectomy**

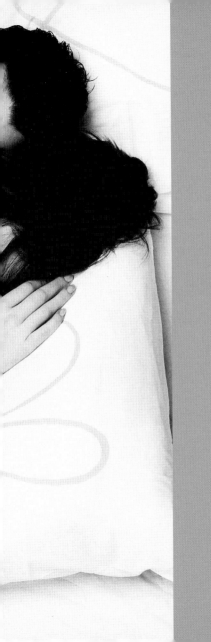

# SURGICAL METHODS

## NO MORE KIDS — THAT'S IT!

Surgical methods are used by individuals who are seeking a permanent method of contraception. Reversing these surgeries is usually complicated and costly and may even be impossible in some cases.

Before choosing a permanent method like tubal ligation or vasectomy, it is important that both partners in a couple discuss this step to prevent them from regretting their decision in the future. We will provide you with information to help you decide.

In the 2002 Canadian Contraception Study, surgical sterilization (male and female combined) was the second most frequently used method of contraception following the oral contraceptive pill.

# TUBAL LIGATION DISCONNECTION THE FEMALE WAY

**Who controls the show?**
The woman.

**Does it protect against sexually transmitted infections and HIV?**
No.

**What is tubal ligation all about?**
The two fallopian tubes, which transport the egg(s) after ovulation to the uterus, get disconnected or plugged with a device. It then becomes impossible for the egg to meet up with the sperm. **A tubal ligation is meant to be permanent. Reversing a tubal ligation is difficult, risky, and costly.**

**What makes this method so special?**
- It is one of the most effective methods of contraception offered to the woman.
- It is for women who have completed their families and who do not want any other form of contraception (e.g. IUD, IUS or OC).

**How do I get it?**
You and your partner should discuss your options first. You then need to see a gynaecologist who performs surgery. You can expect a full gynaecological exam and questions to make sure that you will not regret your decision. You will have to sign a consent form.

When discussing this with your partner, keep in mind: A vasectomy, the male sterilization, is a much easier procedure and it involves fewer health risks.

**Possible problems**
Pain, bleeding, nausea following surgery.
The biggest problem is regret. You have to keep in mind that this surgery makes a woman permanently sterile. The reversal is sometimes possible but does not always work out. Discuss it with your partner!

**How effective is tubal ligation in preventing unintended pregnancy?**
99.5% effective.

**Necessary routine**
No routine. You do not have to worry about contraception any more.

## WHAT IS TUBAL LIGATION ALL ABOUT?

It is a surgical procedure that provides permanent contraception. It interrupts the journey of the female egg to the uterus. Tubal ligation (ligation=binding) is also referred to as female sterilization. To be sterile means to be unable to reproduce. **It is mostly chosen by women who have completed their families because it is permanent. The surgery does have risks and reversing the surgery is very difficult.**

### How does tubal ligation work?

During ovulation, an egg leaves one of the ovaries, travels through the fallopian tube towards the uterus, and awaits the encounter of sperm to get fertilized. Tubal ligation blocks both fallopian tubes. This means that the egg cannot travel to the uterus and that the sperm cannot meet up with the egg. The procedure does not affect the daily work of the ovaries. The female cycle with its hormone production, ovulation and menstrual periods, remains the same afterwards.

### How effective is tubal ligation in preventing unintended pregnancy?

Failure rates following tubal ligation are reported over a time period of 10 years following the surgery. They vary between 0.5 and 2.5% depending on the kind of procedure chosen by the physician. Studies have shown that the probability of failure for women sterilized at age 28 or younger is higher than in women who have the surgery past the age of 34.

### Does tubal ligation protect against sexually transmitted infections and HIV?

No. Remember that there is no such thing as a free ticket to a worry-free love and sex life! It is handy to choose a method like sterilization, which effectively protects against pregnancy, but remember that it doesn't protect you from diseases. If you and/or your partner are not mutually faithful to each other, or if you are at risk for STI and HIV, you should use a male or female condom for protection. Practice safer sex: use dual protection.

### How popular is tubal ligation in Canada?

Here are some statistics from the 2002 Contraception Study:

- Tubal ligation was used by 7% of all women in the study.
- Married women (33%) were more likely to have a favourable opinion towards tubal ligation than unmarried women (21%).
- Of women who were planning on using a permanent method of contraception, most (55%) planned for their partner to have a vasectomy. In fact, more men than women were sterilized.

### Tubal ligation may be a good choice for you, if...

- you and your partner are sure that you do not want to have more children or any children at all
- you want a very effective, long-term method
- you want a very private method
- you want a method, which is not related to intercourse
- other (reversible) methods such as hormonal methods or the IUD/IUS are not options for you

### Tubal ligation is not for you, if...

- you are not sure that you want permanent contraception
- you are pregnant
- you have health problems which may be aggravated by anaesthesia
- your partner agrees to have a vasectomy because it is an easier procedure with fewer complications

### What to expect when getting a tubal ligation?

First, the physician who will perform the procedure will ask you questions. Please read the following paragraph to be prepared for some of the questions. It is very important to be absolutely sure that you want a tubal ligation because it is, in principle, a method of no return! You will have to sign a consent form.

Second, you will be examined to check whether this procedure can be done for you. The physician will want to find out whether

First of all, if you have a partner, you and your partner should carefully discuss your options to **avoid regretting your choice in the future. With permanent sterilization, it is important that you and your partner have one another's support and agreement before going ahead with the procedure, although you do not need your partner's permission.** The procedure itself is done by a gynaecologist. Ask your family physician, gynaecologist or family planning clinic where you should go.

he or she can easily access the tubes, whether you have any infections, or whether you are pregnant. You will also get information about the possible risks that go along with general or local anaesthesia.

After this first visit you will get the appointment for the surgery. The time between the two visits is very important for you to consider your decision. Here is some support to help you with your decision:

### You have to sit back and think and rethink...
If you are sterilized you will not be able to become pregnant any more. Do you really want this? Here is some food for thought:

- ☐ Will I feel like less of a woman if I am sterile?
- ☐ Is there a possibility that my partner could change his mind and suddenly want to have another child with me?
- ☐ Is my partner aware of the fact that we cannot have any children or any more children together?
- ☐ Is there a possibility that I might break up with my partner, meet another partner, and want to have a child with him or her?
- ☐ Is my partner in favour of my decision to have a tubal ligation?
- ☐ If one of my children dies, will I want another child?
- ☐ Have I thought about other possible methods of contraception, which are less risky and not as final? (e.g. vasectomy, IUD, IUS)
- ☐ If you do not have a steady partner and want to protect yourself from becoming pregnant keep the following in mind:

**Tubal ligation is not the right contraceptive method for you if you're changing partners. You still need condoms to protect yourself from sexually transmitted infections and HIV.**

Take some time to think about these questions. Discuss them with your partner and be really sure you still want the tubal ligation before you go for it!

### Regret. Better to be sure than sorry!

Studies have shown that regret happens in 5% of cases. Here are the most common reasons why women regret their decision and contact their physicians to get a reversal. Could that happen to you as well?

Read this and check your decision one more time:

- ☐ I was too young (under 30).
- ☐ I had young children, and now that they are grown we want another child.
- ☐ The relationship was not going well.
- ☐ I did not get enough information about it in the first place.
- ☐ I was pushed into it by my partner.
- ☐ I do not feel like a real woman any more.
- ☐ I found a new love and want a child with my new partner.
- ☐ My financial situation has improved and I can afford more children.

### Some words about the surgery itself

There are four kinds of procedures:

1. Operating through a very small incision in the bellybutton. The procedure is called <u>laparoscopy</u> or band-aid surgery. It can be performed under local anaesthesia in some cases. Through this incision, the tubes will be tied, cut, or a clip or ring may be applied to them.

2. Another technique, called <u>transcervical</u>, involves inserting a nickel-titanium and stainless steel coil (Essure®) into the fallopian tubes using a hysteroscope.

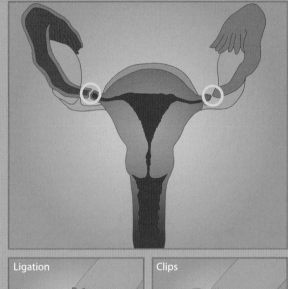

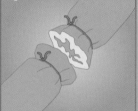
Ligation

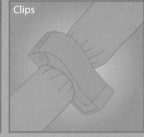
Clips

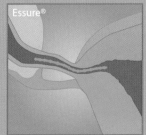
Essure®

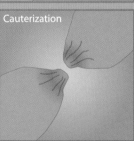
Cauterization

The metal coil blocks the fallopian tubes. This method requires minimal sedation and no surgical incision. The surgeon uses the hysteroscope to enter the uterus through the vagina and cervix. It also allows quick recovery.

3. Operating through a larger incision in your belly. The procedure is called a laparotomy. This also can be performed under regional anaesthesia in some cases. It is less common, but often used when a tubal ligation is requested shortly after delivering a baby.

4. Operating through the vagina. This is called colpotomy and is hardly performed in North America anymore due to higher failure rates and complications.

The choice of the method depends on the physician and on the timing of the surgery. It can be performed after the delivery of a baby, at the time of a therapeutic abortion, or at any other time.

### Precautions after surgery
- No sports or physical strain for at least seven days after the surgery
- If intense pain and high fever occur, contact your physician immediately
- No restrictions on intercourse, unless the transcervical method was used.

Tubal ligation is effective from day one after surgery. With the transcervical method (Essure®) another contraceptive has to be used for 12 weeks until the doctor has made sure that the tubes are blocked.

The recovery period following a laparotomy is longer compared to a laparoscopy or the transcervical method.

# TROUBLESHOOTING

After the procedure there might be some reactions that cause discomfort. These short-term complications vary with the type of surgery performed and the type of anaesthesia used. The most common are:

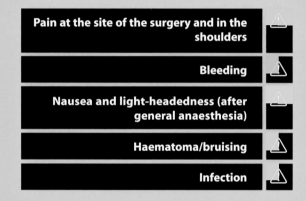

| Pain at the site of the surgery and in the shoulders |
| Bleeding |
| Nausea and light-headedness (after general anaesthesia) |
| Haematoma/bruising |
| Infection |

Studies are ongoing to find out about the long-term complications of tubal ligation. The risk of ectopic pregnancy following a reversal is about 5%. An ectopic pregnancy is a pregnancy at the wrong place, meaning outside the uterus. If signs of pregnancy start showing, you should contact your physician immediately.

**If I ever regret the tubal ligation, is there a chance to reverse the procedure and become fertile again?**

If you had a transcervical procedure performed the chances are next to zero. With the other techniques, yes, there is a chance. But it is much more complicated than the tubal ligation itself and it is very expensive. The probability of pregnancy following tubal ligation reversal is between 52% and 90% and depends on how the surgery was first done, and of course on the skills of the surgeon. There is a 20% higher risk for ectopic pregnancy after reversal surgery.

 **Does it affect my desire, my ability to make love?**

No. Think of the tubal ligation as a mechanical interruption of the transportation route of the eggs. The fact that the eggs cannot travel to the uterus has no effect on your hormones, cycles, periods, desire, lovemaking or ability to reach orgasm. Many women enjoy the freedom they feel after the procedure because they do not have to worry about contraception any more.

**Does it affect my periods?**

Some women have reported changes in their cycles. However, according to studies, cycle changes are not related to the tubal ligation itself. If you were taking the birth control pill prior to having the surgery, your periods were probably very regular before the surgery. After the surgery, when you stop taking the pill, your periods may be irregular initially. They will often become similar to what they were prior to starting the pill.

**IN A NUTSHELL**

# VASECTOMY DISCONNECTION THE MALE WAY

**Who controls the show?**
The man.

**Does it protect against sexually transmitted infections and HIV?**
No.

**What is vasectomy all about?**
The surgery blocks the vas deferens and prevents sperm from entering the ejaculate. The man can still ejaculate when reaching orgasm but the fluid, which leaves the penis during ejaculation, does not contain any sperm.

The man is infertile and cannot make a woman pregnant any more. **A vasectomy is considered permanent because a reversal is difficult and costly.**

**What makes this method so special?**
- It is the most effective method of contraception offered to the man.
- It is an easy procedure with very few known side effects.
- It is a permanent method.
- It is a good alternative if the female partner cannot use hormonal methods or the IUD/IUS.
- It relieves the woman from the contraceptive burden.

**How do I get it?**
You have to discuss this decision with your female partner. You have to see a urologist, a family physician, or go to a family planning clinic. The physician will examine you and will find out whether you are a candidate for this procedure. **After the procedure there is a three-month period during which time you can still have sperm in your ejaculate.** Until you have your follow-up visit you have to use another form of contraception.

**Possible problems**
Certain discomforts like swelling following surgery. The biggest problem is regret. You have to really think about it and the consequences, and keep in mind that it is permanent. The reversal does not always work out. Think and discuss with your partner!

**How effective is vasectomy in preventing unintended pregnancy?**
99.85-99.9% effective.

**Necessary routine**
No routine. You do not have to worry about contraception any more.

## WHAT IS VASECTOMY ALL ABOUT?

Vasectomy is also referred to as male sterilization. To be sterile means that you cannot reproduce any more. The surgery blocks the right and left vas deferens to prevent the journey of the sperm into the ejaculate (fluid which leaves the penis during ejaculation). The man can still ejaculate but there is no more sperm in the ejaculate, meaning that he cannot make a woman pregnant.

**It is considered a permanent method of contraception chosen mostly by men who have completed their families because it is very difficult and costly to reverse the surgery.**

### How does vasectomy work?
You remember our anatomy chapter in the beginning of the book? It takes sperm around 70 days to mature. The mature sperm finally reaches the vas deferens. Sperm is stored in the vas deferens until ejaculation occurs. During ejaculation, sperm and liquid from the seminal vesicles make a mix that is called semen. When the vas deferens is cut sperm cannot get into the ejaculate.

There are different techniques to do this and your physician will tell you about the choices you have.

### How effective is vasectomy in preventing unintended pregnancy?
Pregnancy rates following vasectomy vary from 0.1 to 0.2%. It is, apart from female sterilization (called tubal ligation) and of course abstinence (no intercourse), the safest method of contraception. Now you might ask why a failure rate is still possible? The answer is simple. After the procedure there is a possibility that the testicular side of the vas finds its way and reaches the distant part of the vas (which was disconnected before).

This complication is called recanalization (meaning a communication reoccurs between the two ends of the vas). A recanalization generally happens within the first three months after surgery in 2.6% of cases. This is why we recommend the use of a backup method between the time of surgery and the check-up visit three months later. The main reason for pregnancies after a vasectomy is the failure to use a back-up method during the three months following surgery.

### Does vasectomy protect against sexually transmitted infections and HIV?
No, it does not protect against sexually transmitted infections and HIV. Everything we have discussed in Chapter 2 on safer sex applies to sex partners who have chosen a vasectomy as well. The exchange of body fluids during intercourse makes bacterial and viral infections possible. **The fact that there is no sperm in the ejaculate after a vasectomy was performed does not mean that there is a lower risk of infecting the partner with an STI or HIV. A condom protects you. Practice safer sex and use dual protection!**

### How popular is vasectomy in Canada?
In the 2002 Canadian Contraception Study, vasectomy was used by 13% of respondents. It is used more often than tubal ligation (7%).

### Vasectomy is a good choice for you, if...
- you and your partner are sure that you do not want to have more children or any children at all
- you want a very effective long-term method, which is safe, easy and not related to intercourse
- you want to relieve your female partner from the contraceptive burden
- your female partner cannot use other methods which are reversible such as hormonal methods or the IUD/IUS
- your female partner is considering a tubal ligation (female sterilization). A vasectomy is easier and has less risk of side effects

**HOW DO I GET A VASECTOMY?**

First of all, if you have a female partner you should discuss this choice with her. **To avoid later regret, it is important to have the support and agreement of your partner for this method more than for any other.** Vasectomies are performed by family physicians or urologists (physicians specialized in treating diseases of the urogenital tract, which consists of the bladder and reproductive organs in men). Contact your family physician or a family planning clinic to get the address of a physician where you can make an appointment.

**Vasectomy is not good choice for you, if...**
- you are not sure that you want permanent contraception
- there is any possibility that you may regret this decision
- you have health problems which may be aggravated by anaesthesia
- you have a local infection
- you suffer from sexual dysfunction

**What to expect when getting a vasectomy?**
First of all, the physician who will perform the procedure will ask you a few questions. Please read the following paragraph to be prepared for some of them. It is very important to be absolutely sure that you want it done because it is a method of no return!

Second, you will be examined to find out whether this procedure can be done. After this first visit you will get the appointment for the vasectomy along with instructions how to prepare yourself for the surgery. The time between the two visits is very important to rethink your decision. Here is some support to help you with your decision:

**You have to sit back and think and rethink...**
After a vasectomy you will not be able to make babies. That's it, finished. Do you really want this? Here is some food for thought:

- ☐ Will I feel like less of a man if I am sterile?
- ☐ Is there a possibility that I could break up with my partner, meet another woman and want to have a child with her?
- ☐ Is my partner aware of the fact that we cannot have any children or any more children together?
- ☐ Is there a possibility that my female partner might change her mind and all of a sudden want to have another child with me?

- ☐ Is my partner in favour of my decision to have a vasectomy?
- ☐ If one of my children dies, will I want another child?
- ☐ Have I thought about other possible methods of contraception which are less risky and not as final?
- ☐ If you do not have a steady partner and you consider a vasectomy to protect yourself from becoming a father against your will, keep the following in mind:

Women do not necessarily believe the man when he says: "You don't need a contraceptive because I had a vasectomy." The woman has no way of verifying this. She will probably insist on another contraceptive.

Vasectomy is not the right contraceptive method if you want worry-free sex while you're changing partners. You still need a condom to protect yourself and your partner from sexually transmitted infections and HIV.

Take some time and think about these questions. Discuss them with your partner and be really sure you still want the vasectomy before you go for it!

### Regret.  Better to be sure than sorry!

Here are the most common reasons why men regret their decision and contact their physicians to get a reversal...Could that happen to you as well? Studies have shown that it happens in 5% of all cases.

Read this and check your own decision one more time:

- ☐ I was too young (under 30).
- ☐ I had young children, and now that they are grown we want another child.
- ☐ The relationship was not going well.
- ☐ I did not get enough information.

- ☐ I was pushed into it by my partner.
- ☐ I do not feel like a real man any more.
- ☐ I found a new love and want a child with her.
- ☐ My financial situation has improved and I can afford more children.

### Some words about the surgery itself

There are two ways to perform it:

1. The conventional way
   The skin of the scrotum is cut with a scalpel, the vas deferens is cut and 1.5 cm on each end of the vas is removed. The open ends are sealed as well as the incision in the scrotum.
2. The no-scalpel vasectomy
   In this method a tiny little cut using a puncture instead of a scalpel is made to go into the scrotum to cut the vas deferens.

Both procedures are performed under local anaesthesia. After the procedure you can go home. The no-scalpel method is associated with fewer complications than the conventional method.

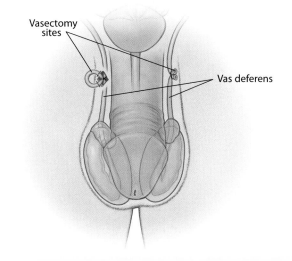

Vasectomy sites

Vas deferens

**? If I ever regret the vasectomy is there a chance to reverse the procedure and become fertile again?**

Yes, there is a chance. But, of course it's a hassle and the chances become slimmer the more time passes after the procedure. Here is a table to tell you what to expect.

## PROBABILITY OF PREGNANCY FOLLOWING VASECTOMY REVERSAL

| Time since vasectomy | Sperm in the semen (%) | Pregnancy (%) |
|---|---|---|
| Less than three years | 97 | 76 |
| 3-8 years | 88 | 53 |
| 9-14 years | 79 | 44 |
| More than 14 years | 71 | 30 |

**? Do I still produce sperm?**

Yes. But since it cannot get out, the body absorbs it.

**? Does it affect my desire, my ability to make love?**

No. Think of the vasectomy as a mechanical interruption of a canal that transports sperm. This canal has nothing to do with sexual desire, ejaculation, or getting an erection. The man will still ejaculate but there won't be any more sperm in the ejaculate. It looks the same, though.

Many couples even report an improved sex life because they do not have to worry about unintended pregnancy any more. And it frees the woman from looking after contraception.

## Precautions after surgery

- No sports or physical strain for seven days after the surgery
- No intercourse for five days
- If strong pain and high fever occur, contact your physician immediately
- **Use another method of contraception for three months following surgery. There still might be sperm in your ejaculate. It takes at least 15 ejaculations until the tubes are cleared of sperm.**

After this period you have to go for a check-up. A sperm count will be done in the laboratory to find out whether your ejaculate is sperm-free and the vasectomy was a success.

# TROUBLESHOOTING

After the procedure there might be some reactions that cause discomfort. Common reactions include:

| | |
|---|---|
| **Pain at the site of the surgery** | ⚠ |
| **Swelling** | ⚠ |
| **Dizziness during the surgery** | ⚠ |
| **Haematoma (1-10%)** | ⚠ |
| **Infection (0.4-16%)** | ⚠ |

Studies are ongoing to find out about any long-term complications from a vasectomy. There have been concerns that a vasectomy might increase the risk of getting a cardiovascular disease, cancer of the testes and the prostate. As of today, no connection between vasectomy and cardiovascular disease or cancer of the prostate could be found.

In the 2002 Canadian Contraception Study, natural methods (including no sex at all) were used by 8% of respondents.

This chapter is about the following methods:

**Abstinence**

**Withdrawl**

**Fertility Awareness**

# NATURAL METHODS
## KNOWING YOUR BODY

"Natural" contraceptive methods do not rely on contraceptive devices, medications or surgical procedures. The effectiveness of the methods in this chapter depends entirely on you and your partner's skills and talent! All natural methods depend on cooperation between partners and they are basically the cheapest methods in the world.

If you get serious about any of the following methods, you and your partner will benefit from them in many ways. They help you to better understand your bodies and maybe even your relationship!

The following information should help you to find out whether you are ready for this! We will talk about:
- Abstinence
- Withdrawal
- Fertility Awareness

For natural methods to work, you have to:
- Understand your body
- Understand how fertilization works
- Understand the female cycle
- Understand and accept unplanned pregnancy
- And the most important thing: you have to be disciplined and you have to have a partner who also supports the method, understands what it is all about, and who is disciplined as well.

This is not for the spontaneous amongst you! If spontaneity is key for you in your sex life please forget about natural methods of contraception. They are definitely a no-no for you!

# ABSTINENCE

## What is abstinence all about?

People who abstain from sexual intercourse or other sexual activity as a way of avoiding pregnancy are said to be using abstinence.

Some people make a conscious decision to avoid sexual intercourse or sexual activity and this is called "abstaining from sexual activity". These people may not want to engage in sexual activity right now for religious, cultural, or other individual reasons, or because they are not ready to have intercourse in their relationship yet.

Abstinence protects against **unplanned pregnancy**. Not having sexual intercourse means the penis does not enter the vagina, hence no sperm can enter the vagina. If a man ejaculates near the vaginal opening, there is a chance that sperm might get in. Abstinence may thus also include avoidance of sexual activities that carry this risk.

Abstinence protects against **unplanned pregnancy and STI/HIV infections** if intercourse is avoided <u>and also</u> risky sexual activities which allow

- skin to skin contact in the genital area and the mouth and
- the exchange of body fluids such as pre-ejaculatory fluid, semen, blood, saliva and vaginal fluid are avoided.

## Does it protect against sexually transmitted infections and HIV?

Yes, if used correctly.

## How do I get it?

In theory, it is free and available to everybody but for many people it may be a challenge to negotiate the use of abstinence with their partners.

## How effective is abstinence in preventing unintended pregnancy?

This can be a very effective method.

## What benefits might people find in abstinence?

- Partners in a relationship have to talk and they have to agree on abstinence and what it means to their partnership.
- Abstinence encourages the use of other pleasuring techniques which might enrich the sexual relationship.
- It is a way to test understanding and feeling for each other at the beginning of a relationship.
- It is used in combination with fertility awareness methods which require abstinence from intercourse during a woman's fertile days.

## Possible problems

You and your partner may have a different understanding of what abstinence is. Another problem is when you suddenly change your mind in the middle of sex play. Always have a condom handy as a standby!

## Necessary routine

Stick to your chosen method!

## WHAT IS ABSTINENCE ALL ABOUT?

The definition of abstinence used in this book varies with the goal people have in mind when they choose abstinence. The goals may be to avoid:

1. unwanted pregnancy or
2. unwanted pregnancy and STI/HIV infection

People choose abstinence for many reasons:
- Cultural, religious or other personal reasons to delay sexual involvement.
- Practical reasons to avoid pregnancy and/or infection with an STI or HIV.
- Avoidance of fertile days for people who use fertility awareness methods, thus practicing "periodic abstinence".
- Life circumstances such as lack of a partner.

If the goal is to avoid pregnancy contraception **and** to prevent STI/HIV infection, abstinence implies
- no intercourse
- no sexual practice which might lead to an exchange of pre-ejaculatory fluid, semen, blood, saliva and vaginal fluid
- no skin to skin contact in the genital area
- no oral contact with the genitals

Couples who are not at risk of STIs may choose abstinence simply to avoid pregnancy. In that case, abstinence allows for a wider range of sexual expressions, which may include the exchange of body fluids such as sperm during oral sex.

## How does abstinence work?

The penis does not enter the vagina and there is no exchange of body fluids such as

- pre-ejaculatory fluid
- semen
- blood
- saliva
- secretion from the vagina (vaginal fluid)

Strictly speaking, the penis should not get anywhere near the vagina. As mentioned in previous chapters, sperm has the ability to find its way into the vagina if ejaculation takes place at the entrance of the vagina.

When practicing oral sex, you have to be aware of the fact that mouth-vulva and mouth-penis contact can lead to an STI infection. There are also certain STIs like HPV and herpes, which spread by skin to skin contact.

You might ask yourself:

## Isn't abstinence boring?

Well, not really. There are many ways to express love and desire other than intercourse. You might want to find out about pleasuring techniques that are allowed when using abstinence as a method.

Here are some to give you an idea that intercourse is really only a small part of the fun!

- Kissing
- Hugging
- Masturbating
- Massaging
- Rubbing
- Looking at erotic material
- Breast / Nipple stimulation

**Do not let yourself be talked into intercourse by your friends or by your partner if you do not feel ready for it. It might be a good idea to wait for someone very special. It is your choice and it's your body. You are the boss!**

## How effective is abstinence in preventing unintended pregnancy?

It can be very effective if used consistently. Since sex is supposed to be fun and pleasurable, abstinence may not be ideal when you are thinking long-term. It may be quite difficult to stay committed to this method! There is a good chance that you might get carried away when you are intimate with your partner. You might want to have intercourse. In that case it's handy to have a barrier method with you - just in case! It keeps you out of trouble in the long-term. If you have no protection at all the last option is emergency contraception (Chapter 8). And, staying away from drugs and alcohol helps you to keep control.

## Does abstinence protect against sexually transmitted infections?

If you make sure that there is absolutely no exchange of body fluids, abstinence does protect you against STIs and HIV. For example, mouth-to-penis (fellatio) contact can transmit gonorrhea, syphilis, hepatitis B, herpes simplex virus and chlamydia. Mouth-to-vulva contact (cunnilingus) has been shown to transmit herpes and syphilis. Dry latex or flavoured condoms and the use of a dam can be used to prevent transmission.

## Abstinence may be an option for you, if...

- you want to be protected against pregnancy, STIs and HIV
- you want to delay sexual activities
- you are not sure about the state of your relationship
- you do not want to make an appointment with your doctor
- you want a method of contraception that guarantees no side effects

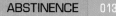 

## Abstinence is not for you, if...

- you are not sure about this choice
- your partner is against it
- you get lots of pressure from your partner or your peers to have sex and you are not sure you can stay firm in your decision to practice abstinence

### What to expect?

Like everything in life, your relationship might change and both of you might want to have intercourse. Then you have to consider another way of reducing the risk of pregnancy and STI/HIV transmission.

To be on the safe side you might want to have condoms with you in case you change your mind in the middle of sex play.

### Where do I get it?

No consultation, no prescription needed!

You have to talk to your partner about it. It is very important that both of you support this method. Imagine your partner tries to talk you into intercourse every time you make love. Then it is just a question of time before the method fails.

## TROUBLESHOOTING

**If passion takes over**

Well, with all the willpower in the world there might be situations when you have intercourse although you wanted to practice abstinence. As mentioned before...it is always wise to have a barrier method handy. If you had unprotected intercourse please refer to the emergency contraception chapter.

**IN A NUTSHELL**

# WITHDRAWAL

**Who controls the show?**
The man and woman together.

**Does it protect against sexually transmitted infections and HIV?**
No.

**What is withdrawal all about?**
The male partner withdraws the penis from the vagina before ejaculation.

**What makes this method so special?**
- It requires self-control.
- It needs practice.
- It requires that both partners cooperate.
- It is a great method when no other methods are available (better than nothing!).

**How do I get it?**
You have to talk to your partner about it. We also highly recommend that you practice with a condom first especially if you and your partner have not been together long.

**Possible problems**
- Inexperience of both partners.
- No control over time of ejaculation.
- Frustration because of the interruption.

**How effective is withdrawal in preventing unintended pregnancy?**
73-96% effective.

**Necessary routine**
Stay disciplined.

## WHAT IS WITHDRAWAL ALL ABOUT?

Withdrawal is a method that is called by its Latin name, "coitus interruptus", interrupted intercourse. You stop the action before it's finished!

It does not offer great protection against pregnancy but it is better than no method at all! In fact, it is more like a risk-reduction strategy than a contraceptive. When you get stuck in a situation when you and your lover want to have sex and you have no method handy... use this one!

### How does withdrawal work?
The man draws the penis out of the vagina and away from the entrance of the vagina (vulva) before ejaculation occurs. This way he prevents sperm from entering the vagina and sperm cannot meet the female egg for fertilization.

### How effective is withdrawal in preventing unintended pregnancy?
Not very effective. There are two reasons why this method is unreliable:
1. This method is entirely based on willpower and practice.
2. There might be sperm in the pre-ejaculate of the erect penis, which gets into the vagina before the penis is withdrawn.

Some studies have shown a failure rate of 4% during the first year of use among users who applied the method perfectly. Typical use had a failure rate of 27%.

### Does it protect against sexually transmitted infections and HIV?
No. Withdrawal only prevents the semen from getting into the vagina. The man is not protected because the penis is exposed to the fluids inside the vagina during intercourse.

The woman is not protected because the vagina is exposed to the pre-ejaculate, which can lead to an STI or HIV infection.

### How popular is withdrawal in Canada?
In the 2002 Canadian Contraception Study, withdrawal was used by 6% of respondents.

### Withdrawal is a good choice for you, if...
- no other method is available
- both you and your partner are free of STIs and HIV
- you are mutually faithful to each other and you can trust each other
- the male partner is used to this method and has not experienced any failures
- you both agree on this method and cooperate accordingly
- you can live with a certain risk of getting pregnant

### Withdrawal is not for you, if...
- there is an STI/HIV risk
- you are looking for a long-term, effective method with almost zero risk of becoming pregnant
- you and your partner get carried away easily during lovemaking
- the male partner cannot anticipate orgasm and ejaculation
- you had previous failure with this method
- you consider withdrawal to be an interruption of lovemaking

### Where do I get it?
You have to talk to your partner about it. It is very important that both of you support this method. Withdrawal can be frustrating at times because it interrupts the sex play.

# TROUBLESHOOTING

The effectiveness of this method is highly dependent upon the cooperation of both partners.

| **Pulled out too late** ⚠ |

This is the most common reason for failure of this method! Don't panic! You can use emergency contraception.

| **Frustration** ⚠ |

Frustration might be an issue. The withdrawal method needs practice to be acceptable for both partners. Both of you have to learn to continue pleasuring each other after the penis has left the vagina in order not to make the withdrawal a break-off point during your sex play.

| **Inexperience** ⚠ |

A word of caution to the woman: If you are in a new relationship and your partner says that he is an expert in withdrawal, you should use a condom anyway. You have to get used to each other and to each other's reactions first. To rely on the withdrawal method at the start of a new relationship is like playing with fire.

## What to expect?

Like everything in life your relationship might change and both of you may want to stop the withdrawal technique. Then you have to consider another method of contraception and protection against STI and HIV.

To be on the safe side you might want to have condoms or other barrier methods with you in case you change your mind while having sex.

Do you know why withdrawal is also called the "basketball technique"?

**The answer is: Because he dribbles before he shoots!**

# FERTILITY AWARENESS

**Who controls the show?**
The man and the woman together.

**Does it protect against sexually transmitted infections and HIV?**
No.

**What is fertility awareness all about?**
The woman keeps track of her monthly cycle by taking her temperature, by checking the vaginal mucus or by tracking other information in a calendar. The idea behind all these methods is to find a pattern behind the individual cycle to predict when the woman is fertile. During the fertile period, the partners have to abstain from intercourse or use another method of contraception.

**What makes this method so special?**
- It requires knowledge and self-control.
- It helps you understand your body and your cycle.
- It requires that both partners cooperate.
- It can also be used to actually plan a pregnancy when you are ready for it.

**How do I get it?**
You have to talk to your partner about it. This method needs the cooperation of your partner. You also have to get more information than this book provides.

**Possible problems**
Lack of knowledge and events which disturb your cycle (illness, stress, peri-menopause, adolescence).

**How effective is fertility awareness in preventing unintended pregnancy?**
75% effective.

**Necessary routine**
Track the cycle and signs of fertility on a daily basis.

## WHAT IS FERTILITY AWARENESS ALL ABOUT?

Fertility awareness is used as a contraceptive method and as a method for those who want to plan a pregnancy. In this book we will concentrate on its use as a contraceptive. Fertility awareness requires knowledge and skills we are not able to address in detail. We recommend further reading. You should contact the closest Canadian Federation for Sexual Health office, a family planning clinic, or Serena, an organization which teaches and provides information on natural family planning. They can provide you with detailed information on fertility awareness methods. Please refer to the address section.

There are various techniques used to practice fertility awareness. The idea behind all these techniques is to determine the fertile days in the woman's cycle. With the knowledge of this fertile time period, intercourse can be avoided or another method of contraception can be used. This group of methods is also called "periodic abstinence".

## How does fertility awareness work?

You have to learn when your fertile days are and abstain from intercourse or use other methods of contraception during this fertile period. The method requires knowledge and discipline.

## What are the principles of fertility awareness?

1. The period starts 14 days after the egg is released from an ovary (ovulation).
2. The female egg lives for 1 day only.
3. Sperm can survive 3 days in the woman's body and can fertilize an egg during this time.
4. Fertilization can therefore happen days after intercourse.
5. The "safe days" during which a woman cannot conceive are from day 2 after ovulation until the new period starts.

Keeping these principles in mind, guess what the big challenge is? To find out when ovulation happens during the cycle.

## Here are the methods to determine the fertile days:

### A. Calendar Method

Idea behind this method: When you keep track of your cycle using a calendar for a few months, you will begin to see a pattern developing. This pattern allows you to determine a time frame when ovulation occurs each month. You simply calculate: The shortest cycle minus 20 days (example: 26 − 20 = 6), the longest cycle minus 10 days (example: 28-10=18). This calculation gives you a window between day 6 and day 18 of the cycle during which time you must abstain from vaginal intercourse or use a contraceptive.

### B. Basal Body Temperature Method

Idea behind this method: Body temperature rises on the day of ovulation and stays 0.5 degrees higher two days after ovulation until menses. The woman has to keep track of her temperature using a special basal body temperature (BBT)-thermometer and mark the readings in a calendar. You will see a pattern developing.

### C. Ovulation or Billings Method

Idea behind this method: The mucus in the cervix becomes slippery, elastic and clear as ovulation approaches. The quality of the mucus changes after ovulation. The woman has to insert her fingers in the vagina and check the quality of the mucus to determine the time of ovulation.

### D. Symptothermal Method

Idea behind this method: It uses the principles of methods B and C. Using a calendar, the woman keeps track of her temperature and the changes of the vaginal mucus. Also, she has to learn to detect changes in the position of the cervix.

### E. Ovulation Predictor Kits

These kits are available in the drugstore and help to predict when ovulation occurs. They test the urine for the presence of a hormone, which shows that ovulation will occur shortly. These are generally used by women who want to conceive. They are also a great tool to help you understand your own cycle.

**F. Breastfeeding**
Idea behind it: Breast-feeding suppresses ovulation. Breastfeeding protects against pregnancy for a period of 6 months after the birth of the baby, provided:

- The woman has not yet had her first period since giving birth.
- The woman breastfeeds the baby regularly and does not use formula in addition to the breast milk.
- There is no more than a four hour delay between feeds during the day, and six hour delay at night.

This method has been shown to be effective in 98% of all cases.

## How effective are fertility awareness methods in preventing unintended pregnancy?

Not very effective. Studies have shown that 25% of users became pregnant within the first year of using one of the fertility awareness methods.

If you are willing to invest time and effort fertility awareness can be quite effective. With perfect use the failure rate is 9% (calendar method), 3% (ovulation method), 2% (symptothermal method), and 2% (breastfeeding).

## Do fertility awareness methods protect against sexually transmitted infections?

No. Practice safer sex: Use a condom for dual protection against STIs and HIV.

## How popular are fertility awareness methods in Canada?

In the 2002 Contraception Study, fertility awareness was used by 2% of respondents.

## Fertility awareness is a good choice for you, if...

- you are willing to invest some time and effort to become familiar with a fertility awareness method
- you and your partner are willing to respect your fertile days (meaning: no intercourse; otherwise another contraceptive method must be used)
- you want to avoid other methods of contraception
- you want to increase the effectiveness of barrier methods by choosing less fertile days for intercourse
- you enjoy learning more about and "listening" to your body, becoming more aware of your health
- you want a method of contraception with a guarantee of no side effects

## Fertility awareness is not for you, if...

- you just had a pregnancy and/or your cycles are irregular (except for the breastfeeding method, which is indicated for women who just gave birth)
- you need protection against STIs and HIV
- your partner is against it and does not want to cooperate
- you are not willing to invest time to become familiar with a method
- routine is not your cup of tea

## What do I have to expect?

Certain challenges along the way and many questions. For example, if you become ill the whole tracking system will no longer give the right information. The methods only work when you are in good shape and your periods are more or less regular.

If you used a hormonal method before, you have to wait a few months until your natural cycle returns before you start with fertility awareness.

It is basically only recommended when you and your partner can accept the failure of this method!

## Where do I get it?

You have to talk to your partner about it. It is very important that both of you support fertility awareness as a contraceptive method. The best idea is to consult the Canadian Federation for Sexual Health, a family planning clinic, or Serena.

## TROUBLESHOOTING

The effectiveness of this method is highly dependent upon the cooperation of both partners. The woman's job is to keep track of her fertile and infertile days, while the man has to respect her fertile days and accept no intercourse or the use of another contraceptive method during this time.

Possible problems are:

### Stress and illness ⚠️

Stress and illness can change the menstrual cycle. You will have to use another method of contraception until the cycle becomes regular again.

### Age ⚠️

Fertility awareness does not work for adolescents because the cycles are not established and regular. Women in peri-menopause also should not rely on this method because the cycles often become irregular before they stop all together.

### Need for emergency contraception ⚠️

If you had intercourse during your fertile days and you do not want to get pregnant you should consider emergency contraception.

# INTRAUTERINE METHODS

## FOR THE LONG-TERM RELATIONSHIP

Intrauterine methods are unique in comparison to all other methods and devices discussed in this book. The intrauterine device (IUD) and the intrauterine system (IUS) may look like barrier methods but they are different from the methods discussed in chapter 4. The contraceptive action is mainly based on a chemical reaction. Furthermore, while other barrier methods have to be inserted and removed before and after intercourse, the IUD or IUS can stay in the uterus for many years.

# INTRAUTERINE DEVICE (IUD)

### Who controls the show?
The woman.

### What is the IUD all about?
A plastic, T-shaped device with a copper wire. A physician inserts the device into the uterine cavity. The copper wire changes the chemistry in the uterus and destroys sperm. **It is a safe and effective contraceptive for women who are at low risk of acquiring sexually transmitted infections and who want long-term contraception (up to 5 years).**

### How do I get it?
You have to see your family doctor, a gynaecologist, or a family planning clinic.

It usually requires two visits. At the first visit, a history is taken, then a physical exam and STI testing is done. At the second visit, the IUD is inserted.

### How effective is the IUD in preventing unintended pregnancy?
99.2-99.4% effective.

### Does it protect against sexually transmitted infections and HIV?
No.

### What makes this method so special?
- Independent from intercourse.
- Long-term contraception for up to 5 years.
- Reversible.
- No negative impact on fertility after removal.
- Good choice for women who cannot use or do not want to use hormonal methods.
- No effect on breast milk.
- Good alternative to sterilization.
- Good for family-spacing.

### Possible problems
Pain and bleeding after the insertion.

### Necessary routine
No routine necessary. You do not need to think about contraception for 5 years.

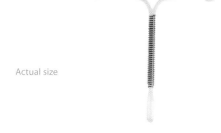

Actual size

## WHAT IS THE IUD ALL ABOUT?

Intrauterine means inside the uterus. The arms of the IUD are flexible and gently rounded to help with insertion and removal. Insertion and removal is the job of a physician.

A copper wire surrounds the T-shaped plastic frame. At the bottom of the IUD there is a polyethylene string. Because the shape of the device mirrors the shape of the uterus, it fits snugly in place without you feeling it.

The IUD is a very effective long-term method of contraception. It can stay in the uterus for up to 5 years. If the IUD is inserted during the late reproductive years (in a woman's forties), it can be left in the uterus until menopause.

The IUD is also used as an emergency contraceptive that can be used within 7 days of unprotected intercourse.

The IUD is a contraceptive option for women who are not at risk or STIs and have a normal uterus.

### Why is that so?

It is better if a woman using an IUD is in an exclusive relationship (one partner only) because she has a higher risk of developing sexually transmitted infections (STIs) and pelvic inflammatory disease (PID) if she or her partner has other sex partners. If she is not in an exclusive relationship, she should use condoms to protect herself against STIs.

### Does it have any non-contraceptive benefits?

Copper IUDs reduce the risk of endometrial cancer.

### How does the IUD work?

The copper wire surrounding the plastic frame creates a chemical environment in the uterus that is unfriendly towards sperm and eggs. The chemical reaction provoked by the copper inside the uterus also destroys sperm so that sperm is not able to travel to the fallopian tubes and fertilization cannot take place. Unlike the oral contraceptive pill, the copper IUD does not prevent ovulation.

### How effective is the IUD in preventing unintended pregnancy?

This method is 99.4% effective if used perfectly. If 1,000 women use this method over a period of one year, 6 women may become pregnant.

### Does the IUD protect against sexually transmitted infections and HIV?

No. The use of a male condom is necessary to be protected. Practice safer sex and use dual protection. The presence of a sexually transmitted infection while an IUD is in place increases the risk of pelvic inflammatory disease and thus the risk of infertility.

### How popular is the IUD in Canada?

In the 2002 Canadian Contraception Study, the IUD was used by 1% of respondents.

# HOW DO I GET STARTED
# WITH THE IUD?

The IUD is an effective contraceptive method right away. From day one of insertion, you are protected from unintended pregnancy.

The insertion can be done at any time during your menstrual cycle. Some physicians prefer to insert the IUD during a woman's menses to rule out pregnancy.

If you have just given birth, you should wait 6 weeks. The IUD is also an effective emergency contraceptive. If it is inserted within 7 days of unprotected intercourse, it can prevent pregnancy (Chapter 8). After an abortion, the IUD can be inserted immediately following the abortion procedure.

## How does the insertion work?

Insertion by an experienced physician should not cause more than slight discomfort. Sometimes a local anaesthetic in the cervix is used. Before inserting the IUD, your doctor will gently slide a speculum into the vagina in order to see your cervix. After that, the depth of the uterus will be measured to find the correct position for the IUD. Using an insertion tube the doctor will then gently slide the insertion tube through the opening in your cervix into the uterus. When it is in place, the arm will open up and form the T-shape.

## The IUD may be a good choice for you, if...

- you have a steady sexual partner (you are faithful to him, he is faithful to you)
- you want a long-term reliable method
- you want to practice "family-spacing"
- you have had failure with other methods in the past (you cannot remember to take a pill daily or you tend to forget to have barrier methods with you)
- you are breastfeeding (the IUD has no effect on breast milk)
- you have completed your family and seek an alternative to tubal ligation
- you have a problem with hormonal methods

## The IUD is not for you, if...

- you are pregnant
- you change sexual partners frequently
- you have an infection or inflammation in your pelvic organs
- you suffer from diseases, which weaken your immune system
- you have bleeding from the vagina which is not related to your period
- you have cervical or endometrial cancer
- you have allergies to the material the IUDs are made of, e.g. copper

## Where do I get an IUD?

You need to make an appointment with your family doctor, a gynaecologist, or at a family planning clinic. Not all physicians insert IUDs so you should ask whether they do when you book your appointment. The doctor will ask you questions about your health and sexual practices (See page 34 - What to Expect On Your Visit) and then perform a medical exam. It is very important to be frank in answering these questions. It is in your own best interest to figure out with your physician whether this is the right method for you. The IUD is not a good idea if you are at an increased risk for sexually transmitted infections or you have already experienced an STI. There are also certain health conditions that might prevent a woman from using an IUD.

Usually at the first visit you will be tested for possible infections. At a second visit, after the results of the tests have arrived, the insertion will be done.

A follow-up visit after six weeks is a good idea. You will be able to ask questions and talk about possible effects that bother you. If everything goes well, you should see your health care provider once a year for your annual check-up.

## What IUDs are available in Canada?

There are two kinds currently available in Canada: Nova-T®, and Flexi-T 300®. You may have heard about the hormonal IUD which is called an IUS. Read about it in the next section.

**FREQUENTLY ASKED QUESTIONS**

 **Does the IUD have an effect on my fertility?**

No. Women who have had their IUDs removed have the same chance of becoming pregnant as women who never used the IUD at all.

 **Do I have to check the strings after each period?**

No. You do not need to check the strings after each period to make sure the IUD is still in place. However you may wish to check the strings from time to time. If you cannot feel them, you should contact your health care provider.

**Can I use the IUD if I never had children?**

Yes, if you are a suitable candidate.

# TROUBLESHOOTING

## Irregular bleeding ⚠

The IUD should not interfere with the normal menstrual cycle because it does not interfere with the hormones in your blood. However, if irregular bleeding occurs, you should contact your physician or family planning clinic. Bleeding irregularities are most common in the first few months of use and usually improve over time. Cramps and slight bleeding following the insertion of the IUD are normal.

## Heavier menstrual bleeding ⚠

Users of copper IUDs have an average of 13 days of bleeding or spotting in the first month after insertion. This decreases to an average of six days after one year of use. Studies have shown that 20% of IUD users have the device removed after one year of use because they experience more pain and heavier bleeding during periods.

## Pain ⚠

This is a rare side effect. Studies have shown that 6% of users are likely to have the IUD removed because of pain after 5 years of use.

## The IUD falls out (expelled) ⚠

In the very rare event that you lose the IUD after insertion, you should see your doctor right away. It may happen to 2-10% of users within the first year.

## Pelvic inflammatory disease (PID) ⚠

At one point there was a lot of talk about an increased risk for PID and IUDs. Recent studies have shown that PID is related to exposure to sexually transmitted infections rather than to the IUD itself.

## Pregnancy complications ⚠

In the unlikely event of a pregnancy with the IUD in place, your doctor should remove the device immediately. If not, there is a greater risk of losing the baby (miscarriage) or having a delivery before the baby is fully grown. Birth defects have not been reported with an IUD in place. You might also want to turn to Chapter 8 where we explained the role of IUDs in emergency contraception.

## The partner feels the strings ⚠

Although the strings attached to the IUD are cut short after the insertion, it is possible that the male partner might feel the strings at the tip of his penis during intercourse. If that occurs, speak to your physician.

## Ectopic pregnancy ⚠

An ectopic pregnancy is a pregnancy that happens out of place, meaning that the fetus grows somewhere other than in the uterus, most likely in the fallopian tubes. If you become pregnant with an IUD in place, there is a greater risk that this could be an ectopic pregnancy. This is an emergency situation and you should seek medical help immediately, especially if you are having considerable pain.

# INTRAUTERINE SYSTEM (IUS)

**IN A NUTSHELL**

### Who controls the show?
The woman.

### What is the IUS all about?
Mirena® is a plastic, T-shaped intrauterine system which prevents pregnancy by slowly releasing small amounts of the sex hormone levonorgestrel into the uterus. A physician performs the placement of the device. **It is a safe and effective contraceptive for women who are at low risk of acquiring sexually transmitted infections and who want long-term contraception for up to 5 years.**

### How do I get it?
You have to see your family doctor, a gynaecologist or a family planning clinic. It usually requires two visits. At the first visit, a history is taken, then a physical exam and STI testing is done. At the second visit, the IUS is inserted.

### How effective is the IUS in preventing unintended pregnancy?
99.9% effective, comparable to sterilization.

### Does it protect against sexually transmitted infections and HIV?
No.

### What makes this method so special?
- Long-term contraception for up to 5 years.
- Good reversible alternative to sterilization.
- Good choice for women who suffer from heavy, painful menses.
- No effect on breast milk.
- No negative impact on fertility after removal.
- Good for family-spacing.
- Independent from intercourse.

### Possible problems
Pain and bleeding after the insertion.

### Necessary routine
No routine necessary. You do not need to think about contraception for 5 years.

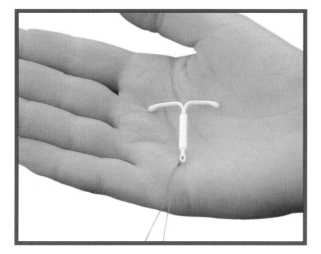

## WHAT IS THE IUS ALL ABOUT?

The intrauterine system (IUS) is a special form of intrauterine contraception because it releases a progestin hormone into the uterus. Mirena® prevents pregnancy by reducing the normal monthly thickening of the lining of the uterus and by thickening the cervical mucus which prevents passage of sperm through the cervix. The IUS is a contraceptive option for women who are not at risk for STIs and who have a normal uterus.

### Does it have any non-contraceptive benefits?
Heavy bleeding during menses (menorrhagia) improves with the use of the IUS (effect of the progestin). Studies have shown a reduction in blood loss of 74-97%. Menstrual pain can also be reduced with the IUS.

### How effective is the IUS in preventing unintended pregnancy?
This method is 99.9% effective and thus comparable to male sterilization.

### Does the IUS protect against sexually transmitted infections and HIV?
No. The use of a male condom is necessary to be protected. Practice safer sex: use dual protection. The presence of a sexually transmitted infection while an IUS is in place increases the risk of pelvic inflammatory disease (PID) and thus the risk of infertility. However, the incidence of PID among IUS users is less than two episodes per 1,000 years of use, similar to the incidence in the general population.

### The IUS may be a good choice for you, if...
- you are thinking about a hysterectomy because you suffer from heavy, painful periods
- you are a smoker and over 35 years-old
- you want a long-term reliable method
- you want to practice "family-spacing"
- you have had failure with other methods in the past (you cannot remember to take a pill daily or you tend to forget to have barrier methods with you)
- you are breastfeeding (the IUS has no effect on breast milk)
- you have completed your family and seek an alternative to tubal ligation
- you cannot take or cannot tolerate estrogen
- you have a steady sexual partner and low risk of infection

### The IUS is not for you, if...
- you are pregnant
- you change sexual partners frequently
- you have current or recurrent infection or inflammation in your pelvic organs
- you suffer from diseases which weaken your immune system
- you have unexplained bleeding from the vagina which is not related to your period
- you have cervical or endometrial cancer
- you have breast cancer

### Where do I get an IUS?

You need to make an appointment with your family doctor, a gynaecologist, or at a family planning clinic. Not all physicians insert IUSs so you should ask whether they do when you book your appointment. The doctor will ask you questions about your health and sexual practices (See page 34 - What to Expect On Your Visit) and then perform a medical exam. It is very important to be frank in answering these questions. It is in your own best interest to figure out with your physician whether this is the right method for you. The IUS is not a good idea if you are at an increased risk for sexually transmitted infections or you have already experienced an STI. There are also certain health conditions that might prevent a woman from using an IUS.

Usually at the first visit you will be tested for possible infections. At a second visit, after the results of the tests have arrived, the insertion will be done.

A follow-up visit after six weeks is a good idea. You will be able to ask questions and talk about possible effects that bother you. If everything goes well, you should see your health care provider once a year for your annual check-up.

### What IUS is available in Canada?

There is only one product on the market and it is called Mirena®.

### How do I get started with the IUS?

The IUS is an effective contraceptive method right away. From day one of insertion you are protected from unintended pregnancy but it is recommended to wait 24-48 hours before having intercourse.

The insertion can be done at any time during your menstrual cycle but it is preferred to have Mirena® inserted within 7 days from the onset of menstruation. If you have just given birth you have to wait 6 weeks. The IUS cannot be used for emergency contraception.

### How does the insertion work?

Insertion by an experienced physician should not cause more than slight discomfort. Sometimes a local anaesthetic in the cervix is used. Before inserting the IUS, your doctor will gently slide a speculum into the vagina in order to see your cervix. After that, the depth of the uterus will be measured to find the correct position for the IUS. Using an insertion tube the doctor will then gently slide the insertion tube through the opening in your cervix into the uterus. When it is in place, the arm will open up and form the T-shape.

## FREQUENTLY ASKED QUESTIONS

**(?) Does the IUS have an effect on my fertility?**

No. Women who have had their IUS removed have the same chance of becoming pregnant as women who never used the IUS at all.

**(?) Do I have to check the strings after each period?**

No. You do not need to check the strings after each period to make sure the IUS is still in place. However, you may wish to check the strings from time to time. If you cannot feel them, you should contact your health care provider.

**(?) Can I use the IUS if I never had children?**

Yes, if you are a suitable candidate.

# TROUBLESHOOTING

## Changes in bleeding pattern ⚠

Bleeding irregularities are most common in the first few months of use and improve over time. Cramps and slight bleeding following the insertion of the IUS are normal. Frequent spotting or light bleeding in addition to your periods may occur during the first 3 to 6 months. In some cases, you may have heavy or prolonged bleeding during this time. About 20% of users become amenorrheic (stop having their periods altogether) over 5 years. Overall, you are likely to have a gradual reduction in the number of bleeding days and in the amount of blood loss each month.

## Reduction in menstrual blood loss ⚠

Most users experience a reduction in menstrual blood loss of between 74-97%. Studies have shown that 14% of IUS users have the device removed after one year of use because they experience more pain and heavier bleeding during periods.

## No bleeding ⚠

This may be a big relief for many women. Between 16-35% of users will have no more menses after one year of use.

## Hormonal side effects ⚠

Some progestin-related side effects such as acne, breast tenderness, and headache may occur in the first few months of use. Weight gain is usually due to eating habits and lack of exercise.

## Functional ovarian cysts ⚠

Cysts have been reported in up to 30% of users. Usually they resolve spontaneously and no special treatment is necessary.

## The IUS falls out (expelled) ⚠

In the very rare event that you lose the IUS after insertion, you should see your doctor right away. It may happen to 2-10% of users within the first year. The risk for expulsion with the IUS is comparable to that observed with the copper IUD.

## Pelvic inflammatory disease (PID) ⚠

Recent studies have shown that PID is related to exposure to sexually transmitted infections rather than to the IUS itself.

## Pregnancy complications ⚠

In the unlikely event of a pregnancy with the IUS in place, your doctor should remove the device immediately. If not, there is a greater risk of losing the baby (miscarriage) or having a delivery before the baby is fully grown. Birth defects have not been reported with an IUS in place.

## The partner feels the strings ⚠

Although the strings attached to the IUS are cut short after the insertion, it is possible that the male partner might feel the strings at the tip of his penis during intercourse. If that occurs, speak to your physician.

## Ectopic pregnancy ⚠

An ectopic pregnancy is a pregnancy that happens out of place, meaning that the fetus grows somewhere other than in the uterus, most likely in the fallopian tubes. If you become pregnant with an IUS in place, there is a greater risk that this could be an ectopic pregnancy. This is an emergency situation and you should seek medical help immediately, especially if you are having considerable pain.

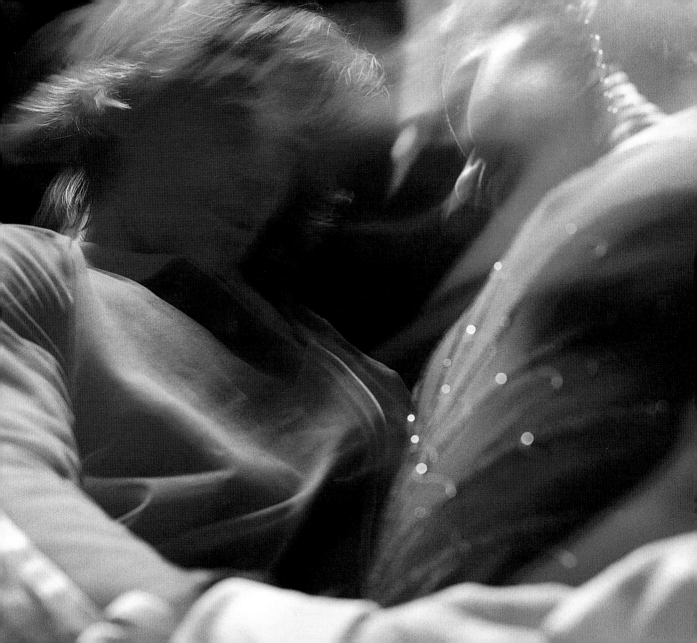

# NO PANIC!

## ALL ABOUT EMERGENCY CONTRACEPTION

You had sex and...in the heat of the moment...forgot all about contraception! Or something went wrong with your barrier method, the diaphragm moved out of place, the condom slipped off... Well, those things happen in life and it's not the end of the world. Taking a bath, using lots of soap, applying vaginal douche or just hoping that you won't get pregnant won't help.

# EMERGENCY CONTRACEPTION

### Who controls the show?
The woman.

### What is emergency contraception (EC) all about?
EC can be used to prevent pregnancy after unprotected intercourse or when a contraceptive method has failed or wasn't used correctly.
- The **emergency OC method** delays or prevents ovulation and works as late as 5 days after unprotected intercourse.
- The **emergency IUD method** creates a chemical environment in the uterus that is unfriendly to sperm and eggs. It works up to 7 days after unprotected intercourse.

### How do I get it?
The **emergency OC method**: go to the pharmacist's counter in any drugstore.

The **emergency IUD method**: you have to make an appointment with your physician a.s.a.p. Make it clear that you need emergency contraception so that you get an appointment immediately.

You can also go directly to a family planning clinic.

### How effective is the emergency OC method in preventing unintended pregnancy?
The emergency OC method prevents 3 pregnancies out of 4.

### Does it protect against STIs and HIV?
No.

### What makes this method so special?
It is a simple and safe way to prevent pregnancy when something goes wrong with your contraceptive or you were forced into having sex. The sooner you take it the more effective it is: so act quickly! Go to the nearest pharmacy or call your physician within 5 days of unprotected intercourse.

### Possible problems
Nausea, vomiting.

### Necessary routine
None because it is used only when needed.

## WHAT IS EMERGENCY CONTRACEPTION ALL ABOUT?

There are two emergency contraceptive methods used in Canada:

1. **The oral contraceptive method (OC):** works within 5 days of unprotected intercourse.
2. **The intrauterine device method (IUD):** works within 7 days of unprotected intercourse.

## One of Canada's best kept health secrets

Emergency contraception is one of Canada's best kept health secrets and is therefore seldom used. Its wider use could dramatically reduce unintended pregnancies and abortions. Now you don't even need a prescription to get emergency contraception in Canada.

In the 2002 Canadian Contraception Study, 57% of respondents knew that emergency contraception existed.

EC is also referred to as post-coital contraception, meaning the method is used after intercourse (post-coital) as opposed to other methods which are used before or during intercourse. EC is also known as the "Morning after Pill". This is a bit misleading because this term only includes the oral contraceptive method and this method can actually be used even later than the "morning after". In fact, it works as late as 5 days after intercourse, but studies show that the sooner you take it, the better it works.

EC prevents pregnancy, for example, in the following situations:

- The condom comes off or breaks.
- Your diaphragm/cervical cap goes out of position during intercourse.
- You miscalculated your non-fertile days and didn't use contraception.
- You missed taking some oral contraceptive pills.
- You were forced into sex.
- You and your partner did not use any method at all.

## How effective is the emergency OC method in preventing unintended pregnancy?

The emergency OC method can prevent 3 of the 4 pregnancies that could be expected after one single act of unprotected intercourse. However, your fertility depends on the time in the cycle when the emergency situation occurred. The days surrounding ovulation are the most "dangerous". Generally speaking there is a 25% chance of becoming pregnant when you've had unprotected sex or experienced contraceptive failure. The sooner you take EC after unprotected intercourse the higher the efficacy. Here are some more figures:

| Method | Hours passed after unprotected intercourse before taking EC | | |
|---|---|---|---|
| | **1-24 hrs** | **25-48 hrs** | **49-72 hrs** |
| Plan B | 95% | 85% | 58% |
| Yuzpe | 77% | 36% | 31% |
| | Prevented Pregnancies | | |

## Does the emergency OC method protect against STIs and HIV?

No. If you had unprotected sex, you should take advantage of your emergency to visit your physician or family planning clinic not only to get emergency contraception, but also to discuss STI and HIV testing. This especially applies to women who were forced into sex.

## How popular is the emergency OC method in Canada?

As yet, there are no statistics. The emergency OC method is now directly available from pharmacists, without a physician's prescription, across Canada. British Columbia was the first province to offer EC directly from pharmacists, making it more widely used within the first year of its new status and leading to a reduction in abortions. The same is expected for the rest of the country.

The emergency OC method uses hormones to prevent or delay ovulation and therefore helps to prevent pregnancy. When it comes to timing, sooner is better. It is most effective when taken within 24 hours. If you can't act right away, EC is still an effective option up to 3 days (72 hours). Although its effectiveness declines the longer you wait, it works up to 5 days after unprotected intercourse. This means you have to take the first two pills no later than 5 days after intercourse for it to work. Bottom line: Don't wait, take it as soon as possible.

There are two different products available. Read the package insert before taking the medication.

**1** Plan B® is the only product approved by Health Canada for the purpose of emergency contraception. After unprotected intercourse or after the failure or suspected failure of a method, you take two progestin tablets containing 750µg levonorgestrel each, 12 hours apart. **Recent studies show that taking two tablets of Plan B® at once is as effective as taking them 12 hours apart.**

**2** The Yuzpe Method (named after the Canadian gynaecologist who developed it) is a combination of four oral contraceptive pills. Each tablet contains 250µg of the progestin levonorgestrel and 50µg of the estrogen ethinyl estradiol.

The IUD method can be used for emergency contraception as well as under "normal" circumstances. After inserting the IUD for emergency contraception, it can be left and used as a long-term contraceptive. It is usually used by women who cannot take hormones and who want a long-term and very effective contraceptive. It is also the most effective form of EC. For the IUD method please refer to chapter 7.

The emergency OC method is a "one time" method, which implies that you have to make a contraceptive choice after using it. In this chapter we will concentrate on the emergency OC method.

## Can any woman use the emergency OC method?

The answer is yes, almost any woman.

- If you are already pregnant from a previous act of intercourse, EC is not an abortion agent and will not work as such.
- If you cannot take oral contraceptives because of blood clots or other health conditions you cannot use the Yuzpe method, but you can use Plan B.

## Where do I get the emergency OC method?

You have to go to your pharmacy and get it straight from the pharmacist. You can also call your family physician, gynaecologist or family planning clinic and explain the situation. No physical exam is required. You won't have to worry about your parents being notified and embarrassing questions.

If you want to see your physician, however, this might be a good chance to ask him or her about contraception. Use this experience to think about contraception so you will not run into this panic again.

## Do I have to take a pregnancy test?

No, if you ask for emergency contraception within the 5-day time frame after unprotected intercourse.

You should have a pregnancy test if you do not start your menses within 21 days of taking EC.

## How often can I use it?

EC is a back-up method and is not meant to replace other methods of contraception. However, repeat use does not seem to pose any health risks.

## What is the difference between an abortion and emergency contraception?

An abortion is performed when the egg has been fertilized and already has settled in the lining of the uterus (implantation) forming an embryo. EC is used before implantation and therefore cannot induce an abortion. Once a pregnancy has started, EC is not effective.

# TROUBLESHOOTING

You may experience nausea, vomiting, dizziness or fatigue. Here are some figures to show you what to expect. These effects are due to a relatively high dose of hormones taken in a short period of time. They are much less common with Plan B. These effects normally disappear within a couple of hours but might last up to two days.

| Method | Side effects in % of users | |
| --- | --- | --- |
| | Nausea | Vomiting |
| Plan B | 23.1% | 5.6% |
| Yuzpe | 50.5% | 18.8% |

**Note: The emergency OC method is simple, easy to use and has minimal medical risk. The exposure to drugs is short and side effects do not usually last long.**

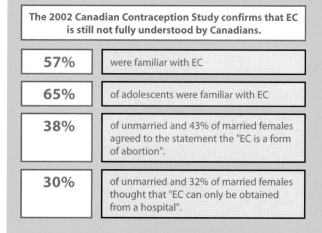

| The 2002 Canadian Contraception Study confirms that EC is still not fully understood by Canadians. | |
| --- | --- |
| **57%** | were familiar with EC |
| **65%** | of adolescents were familiar with EC |
| **38%** | of unmarried and 43% of married females agreed to the statement the "EC is a form of abortion". |
| **30%** | of unmarried and 32% of married females thought that "EC can only be obtained from a hospital". |

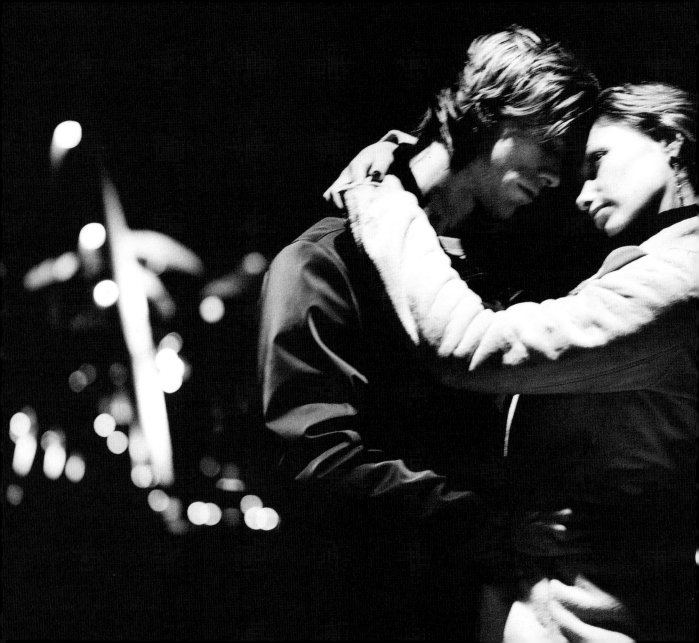

# RETHINK AND ADJUST

## CONTRACEPTION FOR THE PHASES OF YOUR LIFE

A woman can be fertile for over 30 years if we consider that the first period (menarche) is at age 12 and the last period (menopause) is at around 50. Men can conceive children until very old age.

It is one of the big health challenges in our lives to protect ourselves from unintended pregnancy and infections during this long period of fertile years! A contraceptive that suits you and your partner well when you are 20 might be out of the question when you are 40.

**CATEGORIES OF METHODS: A CHAPTER OVERVIEW**

1

2

4

Depending on the relationship with your partner, your health, your age and other facts of your life, you have to rethink and adjust your choice. We want to give you some ideas about the changes you might face and the adjustments you may want to make in the choice of a contraceptive. Your physician or health care provider is your partner in staying healthy and can be a valuable source of information to support you in your choice.

6

7

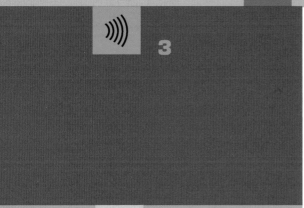

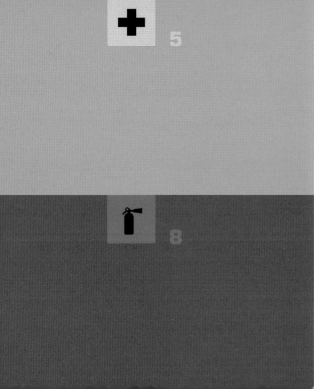

### Adolescence

Your adolescent years are years of exploration and orientation. You will want to check out what sex is all about. You may choose not to have a partner like you might have more than just one partner.

When you make your choice, think of the following: What is effective and easy to use?

You want a very effective method because a pregnancy is probably the last thing you desire and you want protection against STIs and HIV. You also want to preserve your fertility.

### Practice safer sex: use dual protection.

In your adolescent years you have the highest chance of getting infected. HIV and AIDS can kill you. Other STIs, if not treated early, can lead to infertility in men and women. This could be very bad news if you plan to have a family later on. Use a condom (the male latex or polyurethane or the female condom) and you will be protected.

A good choice if you are healthy is to take the pill, patch or ring to protect yourself against pregnancy and to use a condom to protect you and your partner against STIs and HIV.

Hormonal methods used with condoms are very effective methods. Refer to Chapters 3 and 4 and discuss the choices with your health care provider. If you cannot take the pill, progestin-only methods are great, too.

One more thing about the pill: The pill is a great choice for healthy women. However, you have to follow the daily pill-taking schedule. You should also consider the pill as a long-term method of contraception. If you break up with your boyfriend you should not stop taking the pill. Why is that?
- You have to readjust every time to get back into the routine of taking a pill every day
- The body has to adjust every time you start or stop the pill

- The pill offers health benefits apart from being a very effective contraceptive.
- No sex doesn't mean that you should not take the pill. You might find another partner and you will be protected against pregnancy if you keep on taking the pill. Remember that until both you and your partner have tested negative for sexually transmitted infections, you should use condoms.

Since the first edition of **SEX SENSE** in 2000, the contraceptive patch and the ring were introduced. They combine the benefits of the pill with the convenience of once-weekly (patch) or once-monthly (ring) dosing. You do not have to take the hormones daily any more.

We do not want to discourage you from using the sponge, diaphragm and cervical cap. The only problem with these methods is the high risk of failure. They require practice for correct and consistent use.

### After giving birth

If you just gave birth you are facing many decisions. Do I want another child and when? Do I want to breast-feed my baby? We want to give you support for your decision in terms of contraception.

**Breastfeeding** suppresses ovulation. Breastfeeding protects against pregnancy for a period of six months following the birth of the baby, provided:

- The woman has not yet had her first period since giving birth.
- The woman breastfeeds the baby regularly and does not use formula in addition to the breast milk.
- There is no more than a four hour delay between feeds during the day, and six hour delay at night.

If you do not meet these conditions you can become pregnant. The IUD, the IUS and progestin-only contraceptives may be a good choice for women who have given birth and breast-feed because they do not affect the quality and quantity of breast milk.

**If you are not breastfeeding** you can start taking the oral contraceptive pill 3-4 weeks after delivery. Some couples may consider a permanent method of contraception and choose tubal ligation or vasectomy. Barrier methods such as condoms do not have any effect on your system and can be used any time. The diaphragm and cervical cap require refitting after giving birth.

### After a known or suspected contraceptive failure

If you do not want to become pregnant you have to use emergency contraception. The emergency OC method works within 5 days of unprotected intercourse and the IUD method works up to 7 days afterwards. Go to a pharmacy near you. Read more about Emergency Contraception in chapter 8.

### After an abortion

If you had an abortion, you may have had a problem with your contraceptive or you did not use any contraception at all. Depending on the stage of your life you may want to choose a more effective method after this experience. You have to ask yourself how it happened and how you can prevent it in the future.

- Did you have a problem using the contraceptive method?
- Did the method fail?
- Did you use any contraception?

No matter what the answers to the above questions may be, you want to avoid having another abortion in the future so you'll want to make some changes. If you want to have children in the future you may consider a hormonal method of contraception. If you do not want any more pregnancies, a long-term method (IUD, IUS, vasectomy or tubal ligation) might be good for you.

### You are a smoker

Stop smoking! If you are a woman and 35 years of age or older and you do not want to or cannot stop taking the oral contraceptive pill. The pill makes the dangerous habit of smoking even more dangerous. Guys among you: same thing! Show cooperation and stop smoking! If you keep on smoking and you like using hormonal contraception you can switch to any of the three progestin-only methods described in Chapter 3. You may also want to consider the IUD or the IUS.

## Approaching menopause

A woman in her late reproductive years is facing major changes in menopause. She may think about taking hormone therapy to ease menopausal symptoms such as hot flashes, night sweats or vaginal dryness, and protect herself against osteoporosis. In the years before menopause (menopause is considered when one year has passed since the last menstrual period) the cycles become irregular. What many women forget is that they can still become pregnant.

A low-dose oral contraceptive pill offers many health benefits apart from effective contraception. The pill makes periods regular which is a big plus in this stage of a woman's life. Hormonal contraceptives also insure a smoother transition into menopause because the woman herself determines when she has her last period simply by stopping the pill.

If hormonal contraception is not an option, you can choose from the variety of methods presented in this book. The IUS may be a good option for women with unpredictable or heavy periods who need contraception.

## Family spacing

If you and your partner want to use contraception to delay the arrival of a child, the effectiveness of a method may not be the main quality you are looking for. A natural method combined with the use of a barrier method could be a good choice for you. It requires knowledge and practice, qualities that will prepare you for the arrival of a new family member!

Hormonal methods are more effective methods and the return to fertility is usually quite fast when you stop using the method. Excellent alternatives are the IUD or the IUS, provided there is no risk of STIs.

You also may consider that fertility declines with age.

**Effect of age on fertility**

| Age when beginning attempts to conceive | % of women remaining childless |
|---|---|
| 20-24 | 6 |
| 25-29 | 9 |
| 30-34 | 15 |
| 35-39 | 30 |
| 40-44 | 64 |

## In sickness and in health...

When you are sick and take certain medications you have to inform your health care provider and/or pharmacist about your contraceptive method. This especially applies to hormonal methods, which may interfere with the drugs you are taking for treatment of your health problem. The contraceptive may make the medication less effective or the medication you are taking may make the contraceptive ineffective.

## Major surgery

If you have to undergo surgery, which will make you bedridden for a few days, and you are currently taking any form of hormonal contraception (pill, patch or ring), you should probably stop taking it four weeks prior to the day of surgery. There is an increased risk of developing blood clots in your veins when taking hormonal contraception while being immobilized. Don't forget to use another method during this time!

If you had an accident and you undergo emergency surgery you should also stop taking it for a while.

This chapter is all about choices and the adjustment of choices. We can only give you an idea. You have to discuss this in detail with your partner and health care provider to make sure you make the right choice!

# ADDRESSES:
## WHERE TO TURN TO

You need information, support? Here are phone numbers and websites that can help you.

**SOGC: Society of Obstetricians and Gynaecologists of Canada**
Visit the ultimate Canadian website devoted to sexuality education and information.
www.sexualityandu.ca

**Public Health Agency of Canada**
Visit this website for in-depth information on chronic and infectious diseases.
www.phac-aspc.gc.ca

**Canadian Federation for Sexual Health (previously Planned Parenthood Federation of Canada)**
For more information about sexual and reproductive health and rights across Canada, as well as lists of affiliated sexual health centres near you, visit:
www.cfsh.ca

If you do not find the city where you live on the list, call the number near you and ask for the Canadian Federation for Sexual Health branch or clinic closest to you.

*Alberta*
www.plannedparenthoodalta.com
Calgary (provincial) ......................(403) 283-8591
Calgary (local) ...........................(403) 283-5580
Edmonton................................(780) 423-3737
STI/AIDS Info Line.....................1-800-772-2437

*British Columbia*
www.optionsforsexualhealth.org
Vancouver...............................(604) 731-4252
Facts of Life Line.......................1-800-739-7367

*Manitoba*
www.serc.mb.ca
Brandon.................................(204) 727-0417
Winnipeg................................(204) 982-7800

*New Brunswick*
www.fredericton.ppfc.ca
Fredericton..............................(506) 454-6333

*Newfoundland and Labrador*
http://nlsexualhealthcentre.org
St. John's ................................(709) 579-1009

## Nova Scotia

http://www.pphalifax.ca/

Amherst . . . . . . . . . . . . . . . . . . . . . . . . . . . . . . .(902) 667-7500
Bridgewater . . . . . . . . . . . . . . . . . . . . . . . . . . .(902) 543-1315
Halifax . . . . . . . . . . . . . . . . . . . . . . . . . . . . . . . .(902) 455-9656
New Glasgow. . . . . . . . . . . . . . . . . . . . . . . . . . .(902) 755-4647
Sydney. . . . . . . . . . . . . . . . . . . . . . . . . . . . . . . . .(902) 539-5158
Sheet Harbour. . . . . . . . . . . . . . . . . . . . . . . . . .(902) 885-2789

## Ontario

www.ppt.on.ca

Hamilton . . . . . . . . . . . . . . . . . . . . . . . . . . . . . .(905) 528-3009
Kitchener. . . . . . . . . . . . . . . . . . . . . . . . . . . . . . .(519) 743-9360
Ottawa. . . . . . . . . . . . . . . . . . . . . . . . . . . . . . . . .(613) 226-3234
Toronto . . . . . . . . . . . . . . . . . . . . . . . . . . . . . . .(416) 961-0113
Windsor. . . . . . . . . . . . . . . . . . . . . . . . . . . . . . . .(519) 254-3807

## Québec

Contact local CLSCs for family planning services.
The Info-Santé CLSC (Centres Locaux de Services
Communautaires; Local Community Services Centres) Line
is a nursing telephone information and advice service that
responds to health and well-being concerns of the Quebec
population. This service is offered 24 hours a day, 7 days a
week. The number is listed in your local phone book.

Fédération du Québec pour le planning des naissances
(This is not a member of Planned Parenthood)
www.fqpn.qc.ca

## Saskatchewan

Regina . . . . . . . . . . . . . . . . . . . . . . . . . . . . . . . . .(306) 522-0902
Saskatoon . . . . . . . . . . . . . . . . . . . . . . . . . . . . . .(306) 244-7989

## SERENA Canada

For questions regarding Natural Methods contact the
National Secretariat in Ottawa. They can give you the
phone numbers and addresses across Canada.
www.serena.ca
(613) 728-6536
1-888-373-7362

## The Kids Help Phone Line

A service with counsellors for kids from anywhere in
Canada. You can call 24 hours a day, 7 days a week.

1-800-668-6868
Visit the website: http://kidshelp.sympatico.ca

# GLOSSARY

**abortion, spontaneous:** involuntary loss of a fetus before birth.

**abortion, therapeutic:** intended termination of a pregnancy.

**amenorrhea:** no bleeding during the time of the cycle when you normally would expect bleeding (menstruation).

**anemia:** most common form is iron-deficiency anemia caused by the loss of too much blood. Anemia is lack of red blood cells.

**cervical cancer:** cancer of the cervix.

**cervix:** the entrance of the uterus, the passage between uterus and vagina.

**dual protection:** the use of a male or female condom together with another contraceptive method.

**EC:** emergency contraception, methods described in Chapter 8.

**ectopic pregnancy:** an emergency situation, pregnancy outside the uterus, for example in the fallopian tubes.

**endometrial cancer:** cancer (abnormal cell growth) of the lining of the uterus.

**endometriosis:** inflammation of the endometrium. The tissue that makes the lining of the uterus can also grow elsewhere outside the uterus, which can lead to pain during menstruation and more blood loss than usual.

**endometrium:** lining of the uterus.

**estrogen:** female hormone, produced mainly in the ovaries. In its synthetic form (ethinyl estradiol) it is used as a component of oral contraceptive pills.

**failure rate:** term used in studies to describe the effectiveness of a contraceptive method. It is indicated as failure rate for **perfect use** (how effective is the method when it is used consistently and correctly?) and failure rate for **typical use** (how effective is the method when it is not used perfectly?).

**HIV:** Human Immunodeficiency Virus, the virus that causes AIDS.

**HPV:** sexually transmitted Human Papillomavirus, viruses associated with cancer of the cervix.

**IUD:** Intra Uterine Device: a contraceptive described in Chapter 7.

**menopause:** the last menstrual period. Also, phase of a woman's life when estrogen production slows down and fertility comes to an end.

**menstruation:** cyclic bloody discharge from the uterus, also called "period".

**nulliparous woman:** a woman who has never given birth.

**OC:** Oral Contraceptive Pill.

**parous woman:** a woman who has given birth.

**Pap:** stands for Papanicolau stain. A routine test to screen for cancerous cells in the cervix as a prevention of cervical cancer.

**POP:** Progestin-only Pill, a hormonal contraceptive described in Chapter 3.

**pelvic exam:** examination of the inner and outer female reproductive organs described on page 34.

**progesterone:** hormone mainly produced in the corpus luteum (in the follicle from which the egg cell emerged at ovulation).

**progestin:** synthetic female hormone, used for hormonal contraception, either in combination with an estrogen or alone.

**ovarian cancer:** cancer of the female egg-producing organs.

**ovarian cysts:** liquid filled sacs attached to the ovaries that can cause strong bleeding and pain.

**PID:** Pelvic Inflammatory Disease. Inflammation of the inner reproductive organs of a female, which can lead to infertility.

**spotting:** loss of small amounts of menstrual blood outside the normal menstruation.

**STD:** Sexually Transmitted Disease, passed on through sexual contact, also referred to as STI (Sexually Transmitted Infection).

**STI:** Sexually Transmitted Infection, passed on through sexual contact, also referred to as STD (Sexually Transmitted Disease).

**thrombosis:** blood clots that can impair blood circulation.

**speculum:** tool used for the gynaecological exam. It allows the physician to check the walls of the vagina and the cervix.

**unscheduled bleeding:** bleeding from the vagina other than the normal period/menstruation.

**uterus:** also called womb.

**UTI:** Urinary Tract Infection.

**vulva:** female outer reproductive organ, entrance of the vagina.

# INDEX

The Canadian Contraception Guide, 2nd Edition, is based on the
Canadian Consensus Conference on Contraception (2004)
and was developed under the direction of

André B. Lalonde, MD, FRCSC,
Executive Vice-President, SOGC, Ottawa, ON

Sex Sense (1st Edition)

| | |
|---|---|
| Concept, Text, Project Management: | Elke Henneberg, Sutton, QC |
| Editor: | Carol-Ann Savick, Montréal, QC |
| Medical Editors: | Dr. Richard Boroditsky, Winnipeg, MB |
| | Dr. Édith Guilbert, Québec, QC |
| | Dr. Terry O'Grady, St. John's, NL |
| Design: | Student Design Team from the Design Art |
| | Department of Concordia University, Montréal, QC. |
| Art Direction: | Michael Longford, Assistant Professor |
| Design Team: | Tamzyn Berman |
| | Kajin Goh |
| | Tevis Houston |
| | Natacha Vairo |

Sex Sense (2nd Edition)

| | |
|---|---|
| Project Management: | SOGC Communications Division |
| Text: | Elke Henneberg, Sutton, QC |
| Editors: | Elke Henneberg, Sutton, QC |
| | Daniel Morier (SOGC) |
| Copy Editors: | Jacqueline Couture, Ottawa, ON |
| | Mike Haymes (SOGC) |
| Medical Editors: | Dr. Amanda Black, Ottawa, ON |
| | Dr. Richard Boroditsky, Winnipeg, MB |
| | Dr. Édith Guilbert, Québec, QC |
| | Dr. Terry O'Grady, St. John's, NL |
| | Dr. Vyta Senikas (SOGC) |
| Design: | Red Wagon Studio |
| Design Team: | Julie Dorion, Ottawa ON |
| | Jeff Fox, Ottawa ON |